Praise

FACE MASSAGE FOR EVERYONE

T0244890

'Ksenija is proof that skincare can be self-care, but perhaps not in the way you've been led to believe. An hour in her hands is less about the products and all about the technique. Just as a good body massage works to relieve tension, her intuitive strokes can unlock chronically tensed jawlines and reveal sculpted cheeks – and soothe a racing mind just as well.'

ROBERTA SCHROEDER, SENIOR ECOMMERCE EDITOR AT
HARPER'S BAZAAR, ELLE AND ESQUIRE

'I'm so delighted that Ksenija has distilled her key learnings and ethos into something that so many of us can hold, learn from and treasure. This book is a very natural extension of the 360-approach to health that we see in her online presence, where small practices make beautiful moments. I love that she educates in a human, realistic and doable way, meeting anyone that comes across her work where they are. Her teaching is practical and purposeful, and always radiates warm delivery. Reader, you're holding something very special in your hands right now.'

KATIE ENGLAND, CELEBRITY FACIALIST

'A force within the beauty industry: Ksenija has this incredible knack for not only making self-massage approachable for newbies, but also making it fun and joyful at the same time. Many sculpted cheeks and jaw lines around the world have her to thank!'

MARIJKE ADDERLEY, CO-FOUNDER OF BIG BEAUTY

'It's easy to feel the passion Ksenija has for her craft. I've been lucky enough to experience the touch of her hands on my face and it is truly transcendent.'

ESTÉE LALONDE, CREATIVE DIRECTOR AND FOUNDER OF MIRROR WATER

FACE
MASSAGE
FOR
EVERYONE

FACE MASSAGE FOR EVERYONE

A PRACTICAL GUIDE

KSENIJA SELIVANOVA

HAY HOUSE

Carlsbad, California • New York City
London • Sydney • New Delhi

Published in the United Kingdom by:
Hay House UK Ltd, 1st Floor, Crawford Corner, 91–93 Baker Street, London W1U 6QQ
Tel: +44 (0)20 3927 7290; www.hayhouse.co.uk

Published in the United States of America by:
Hay House LLC, PO Box 5100, Carlsbad, CA 92018-5100
Tel: (1) 760 431 7695 or (800) 654 5126; www.hayhouse.com

Published in Australia by:
Hay House Australia Publishing Pty Ltd, 18/36 Ralph St, Alexandria NSW 2015
Tel: (61) 2 9669 4299; www.hayhouse.com.au

Published in India by:
Hay House Publishers (India) Pvt Ltd, Muskaan Complex,
Plot No.3, B-2, Vasant Kunj, New Delhi 110 070
Tel: (91) 11 4176 1620; www.hayhouse.co.in

Text © Ksenija Selivanova, 2025
Photography by Nikita Raja, © Ksenija Selivanova

A catalogue record for this book is available from the British Library.

Tradepaper ISBN: 978-1-4019-8021-4
E-book ISBN: 978-1-83782-282-9
Audiobook ISBN: 978-1-83782-283-6

Interior images: vi: Ksenija Selivanova; 18, 49, 52 Susanne König

10 9 8 7 6 5 4 3 2 1

Printed in the United States of America

*To Mama and Papa: for a lifetime
of nurture and encouragement.*

*And to everyone in my community: you are
the force and motivation behind all my work.*

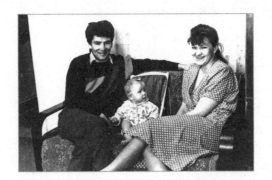

CONTENTS

Contents

INTRODUCTION

Thank you for picking up this book and congratulations on taking the first step towards giving yourself more time and love.

Prioritizing self-care is crucial for our general wellbeing. It's my sacred 'me time.' But many of us lead hectic lives and finding time can be challenging, let alone finding the funds to pay for expensive treatments outside the home. However, self-care needn't be time-consuming or expensive.

You may have picked up this book because, while your friends are getting Botox, you're determined to avoid expensive aesthetic treatments and are looking for more holistic ways to achieve brighter, healthier and younger-looking skin. Or perhaps you find yourself a little sluggish and stuck in a rut, looking for alternative ways to boost your energy and mood. Or maybe you simply heard from a friend how amazing a YouTube video of a face massage made her feel and how much it softened her frown lines, and you got curious. Whatever has brought you here, you've come to the right place.

This book is designed to give everyone, everywhere, the opportunity to get out of a rut and create new positive habits that will benefit all aspects of your emotional, physical and spiritual wellbeing. It's about more than just minimizing lines and wrinkles (though we'll absolutely cover this); I want this book to go beyond the skin and introduce you to the power of rituals to enhance your life in the long term.

My own beauty awakening happened more than 10 years ago, but the roots of that passion go even further back.

Where It All Began

Growing up, my love for skincare came from my mum. In our apartment in a small town called Narva, in Estonia, we'd play beauty salon with whatever ingredients we had to hand: beetroot for blush, cherries for lipstick, used tea bags as eye compresses. I remember her always making peculiar but delicious-smelling concoctions at home that we'd lather over our faces or hair. She'd freeze chamomile tea into ice cubes and use them first thing in the morning instead of washing her face. My mum taught me how to use castor oil on my hair weekly and make wonderful face masks with yogurt and honey. The fundamentals of what I now know to be self-care began here and it was nourishing, giving and holistic.

During my student years, I barely had enough money to buy a face wash, let alone treat myself to a salon facial. Self-massage and home treatments, therefore, became my way to bring a little beauty luxury into my life. I began to incorporate small self-care rituals into my day: massaging my face, dry-brushing my body or mixing a homemade hair mask in my kitchen. It wasn't always flashy, but it was nourishing and nurturing.

This marked the beginning of seeking out alternative ways of caring for my body and, by default, my mind. I strongly believe that beauty is not limited to the reflection in the mirror and, rather, is a reflection of our internal world and wellness — how we truly feel in our skin. And when you look well, you feel well; when you feel well, you look well.

Being a student in a foreign country, I was doing my best to not only fit into a new society, but also manage the expectations placed on me. And there were many times when it all felt too much. But these and other practices allowed me to create a private sanctuary in my own home. My self-care rituals felt safe, serene and loving: my version of meditation that, in turn, helped me process the anxiety and stresses that came with simply existing in the world.

Ever since, I've made it my mission to share my tips and rituals so that others can make self-care part of their everyday lives, too, rather than just a 'treat.' My core belief is that you don't need a lot of money or time to carve out meditative, self-loving moments. It's all about intention and small, daily habits. These moments don't just have to belong to you, they can be shared. I like to say that a bad thing shared is halved, and a good thing shared is doubled. Starting with friends and family, and then taking my routines to social media, I decided I wanted to reach an even wider audience. So, in 2016, I created my channel — *TheMoments* — on

YouTube. I really didn't have any expectations or a predetermined plan. I just started filming face massage tutorials and skincare routines for anyone who wanted to watch. I loved it and, to my surprise, quite a few other people did, too. Today, I can call my subscribers and followers a community and I feel truly honoured and privileged that so many people have shared their journeys with me. It's their support and positive comments that have helped me to keep going, learning, studying and sharing more.

Since starting my YouTube channel, I've trained in face and body massage techniques; qualified as a Pilates instructor, beauty therapist and health coach; embarked on a nutritionist degree; and researched many beauty and wellness methods along the way. In 2021, I opened The Moments Studio London – my little sanctuary where I offer a variety of facial and body treatments. It's become a really special space for me to connect with my clients and grow as a practitioner. When I watch the individuals I treat leave feeling a little lighter and looking at the world a little more brightly, I feel incredibly fortunate.

After receiving countless questions and requests through YouTube, Instagram and in person, I gained a good understanding of the concerns most of us have. Then I took some time to learn and practise techniques and exercises that best suited these concerns. From there, I curated a library of the most effective and easy-to-practise routines, tips and rituals you can do at home, and now I feel so privileged to have been given the opportunity to translate these to print and bring you *Face Massage for Everyone*.

To me, this book offers up my greatest belief and ambition: that everyone, everywhere, should have the opportunity to tap into the luxury of feeling at their best.

How to Use This Book

My intention for this book was always to create a practical, and hopefully inspirational, guide to self-massage – a tool for more self-love and self-care moments in everyone's lives – but how you use it is up to you.

In Part I, we'll explore the fundamentals with a deep dive into the importance of self-care, as well as the many benefits of self-massage – from aiding with lymphatic drainage and smoothing wrinkles to reducing stress. We'll also look at how to get started with face massage, outlining the facial muscles and the best oils and creams to use depending on your skin type (though, as you'll come to see, all you really need for self-massage is your hands!).

In Part II, you'll find my core procedures (*The Basic Routines*) – from the essential warm-up sequence and routines for the morning and nighttime, to routines for different occasions. In Part III, we'll explore a range of routines to address the common feelings and emotions that we experience on a regular basis, while Part IV contains routines to address target areas such as chest and neck lines, jowls and dark circles, as well as offering some guidance on face and eye yoga.

Throughout the book, you'll also find some quick tips from me, as well as some Q&A sections where I answer some of the most common queries I get asked, both in my studio and on social media.

I'd love to think that you will take the exercises from this book and implement them into your daily morning and evening skincare routines. Or instead, you may create a monthly night, where you play with the routines as a group accompanied by laughter, marshmallows and hot chocolate. Or perhaps you'll use the massages as tools when you need a break, a reset or a moment of present calm. And, of course, if your main concern is addressing the visible physical changes we all experience as we age, then there are plenty of massages to target specific areas.

However you decide to use this book, my hope is that you'll see for yourself how transformative — both visibly and invisibly — self-massage can be. Take what you like and need from this book and implement it in your own life.

I hope these pages will serve as a resource you can turn to at any time. I'm excited that you're embarking on this journey, and I'm here with you every step of the way.

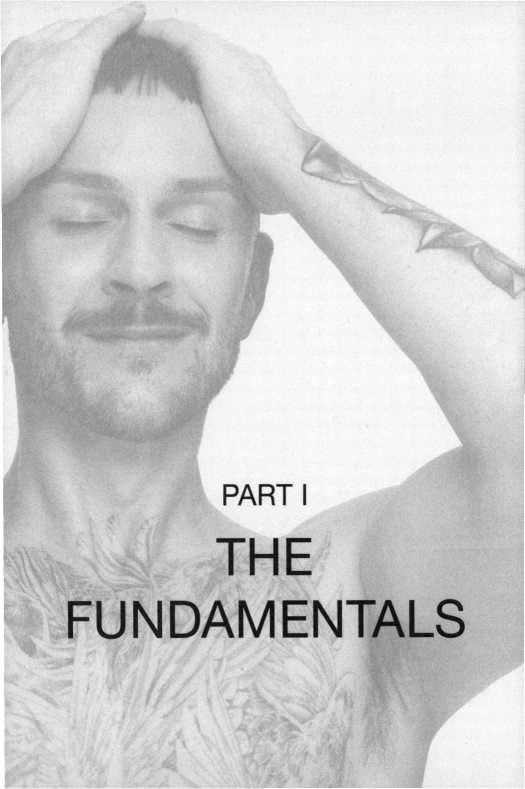

PART I

THE FUNDAMENTALS

The Importance
of Self-Care

We often see the term 'self-care' in magazines and across social media, but what does it really mean and why does it play such an important part in our lives?

I believe that all of you reading this book are giving, caring and loving individuals – we give, we love and often we ask for little in return, but that can be draining. Self-care is about countering that and establishing behaviours and habits that have a positive effect on our wellbeing. It's about taking proactive steps to maintain and improve our physical, mental and spiritual wellness, because if we neglect one, the others will inevitably suffer.

I truly believe that self-care is as individual as our food preferences. One size really does not fit all when it comes to establishing consistent routines that can shift our moods and even the course of our lives. If dancing alone to 'Mr Brightside' in an empty apartment is not what fills your positive energy cup (though, have you tried it?) or the idea of sitting in the lotus position visualizing your chakras triggers an immediate eye-roll, I get it! And if that's the case, it's totally okay! What's important is finding what fills your cup – because, as the saying goes, you can't pour from an empty cup.

Many of us lead busy lives and don't always have the time or energy to commit to high-effort self-care activities, but there are so many ways to practise self-care on a daily basis through smaller activities that can have a big impact, including:

- **Nature.** Just the simple act of taking off our shoes and standing on the grass for five minutes has amazing benefits. Whether it's a walk, a run or sitting down under a tree, just get outside.

- **Meditation or breathwork.** Practising unconditional presence and turning inwards can open up our horizons and peel off the layers of our conditioning, and the patterns and habits we fall into. This can be guided (there are lots of guided meditations and breathwork practices accessible online) or practised solo.

- **Unplug when you can.** This is so much easier said than done, but assigning a specific time and maybe even areas of your home as 'no-device' times and places can bring us back to the present and help turn our attention inwards.

- **Set boundaries.** We all have a bright, burning flame inside of us – it's our spirit, our soul, our power – and we want to surround ourselves with people who protect that flame, who encourage its strength. However, there are people who will constantly try to extinguish your flame. Set boundaries with people who don't make you feel good. Limit time with friends, family and colleagues who make you feel anything less than yourself.

- **Move your body** and schedule workouts that you'll enjoy. When people tell me that they don't like exercising, I always say they just haven't found their workout yet. Find the discipline that works for you; for me it's Pilates, but for you, it might be yoga, badminton, calisthenics, swimming, gardening or silent disco. The important thing is to find a physical activity that you enjoy. Any movement will release happy hormones.

As you can see, you have countless choices of how you can include self-care into your life – from meditation and yoga to ecstatic dancing – and I support and love all of these. But what if I told you that self-massage provides the benefits of them all combined?

Let me explain. What is the core of meditation? Being present. In yoga, it's all about a physical and spiritual practice energizing the body and mind. Ecstatic dancing releases feel-good endorphins and gives us a boost of joy. As we'll explore in the next section, self-massage does all of that – and more.

The practice of massage has evolved over the years and new techniques are always being developed – now, you can get anything from a wooden hammer massage to an intra-oral massage, inside your mouth (I'm a big fan of the latter by the way). For me, self-massage is so much more than a physical release – it's a perfect way to tap into a calmer, happier way of being.

Self-massage is one of the most incredible acts of self-kindness and love. I adore this quote by Michelangelo: 'To touch is to give life' – I couldn't agree more. Touch is our primary language of compassion, trust and safety. There have been hundreds of studies that prove the incredible emotional and physical benefits of touch – it can reduce pain, enhance immune function, alleviate anxiety and stress, improve sleep and reduce fatigue. So even when we can't receive it from others, it's essential to give it to ourselves.

Self-massage provides us with an opportunity for self-healing, as well as improving our day-to-day lives. It does require consistency and dedication, but luckily the positive changes and effects won't leave you waiting long, so it's easy to stay on course. One of the easiest ways to turn self-massage into a regular habit is to incorporate it into your daily routine as a ritual.

Let's Talk About Rituals

There are a lot of things we do on a daily basis simply to get them done – these are our habits. And then there are actions that can spark positive emotions, as well as reward us with physical benefits. This is where rituals come in. They are the shapeshifters, the powerful force that can wash away what is not serving us well and present us with a slightly cleaner slate to move forwards with our day. And, when performed regularly, they have a positive effect on our life.

I'm a true believer in rituals. Over the years, I've developed a few myself and have also adopted others from fellow humans and different cultures. The beauty of rituals is that they're completely individual experiences.

I don't think I was conscious of rituals in my daily routine for many years, but let me take you back to 2007, when I first understood the importance and deeper meaning of rituals.

I spent my late teens studying at university in Finland. Even though it wasn't a very distant move, coming as I do from Estonia, there were some cultural differences and rituals that at first appeared odd to me, but then became something I embraced and very much looked forward to. I studied International Business and attended many lectures on marketing, international finance and accounting (that last part I was truly terrible at). More than 10 years after my graduation, I couldn't tell you exactly what I learned in those three years, but I will tell you about a ritual that's stayed with me ever since.

If you've ever lived in Scandinavia or spent some time there, you might have heard of *fika*. At its simplest, *fika* is a break for coffee and a pastry, which can be had indoors or in the woods, during office hours or after work. But, in reality, it's so much more than that.

For many of us, the idea of 'coffee and a pastry' during a work day means a quick trip to a coffee shop that can leave us with a burned mouth from trying to down the drink too quickly and slight indigestion from a barely chewed croissant. *Fika* is anything but that. It's a state of mind. A ritual. Something you can't experience by yourself. Everyone involved in this ritual takes time to pause, connect, enjoy some coffee, reset and only then continue with their day.

So, just imagine a 17-year-old me in a foreign country, during my first week at university, on my first break after a lecture, watching the Finnish students and teachers pour out of the auditoriums and head to the cafeteria. And here began the lovely buzz of talking, plate-clinking and coffee-pouring. People flocked together to catch up, listen, connect and simply step away from whatever had happened before and what might come after. At first, I couldn't understand why they did this but, as time went on, I was one of the first out the door to make my way towards a cinnamon bun and to enjoy the ritual of *fika*.

Don't get me wrong, I'm still not on board with coffee (especially the brown liquid that came from a thermos they used to drink lots of in my university in Finland), but I'm very much on board with taking a break with your companions and, in return, for yourself; nourishing your mind with a ritual that brings you to the present moment and evokes positive emotions, acting as an anchor or even a positive shift in your day.

A ritual is anything you make of it. Maybe it's a particular way you prepare your coffee in the morning. Maybe it's a stroll in the park at exactly 3 p.m.

every Wednesday. A ritual is anything that we do with intention and presence. It can be a weekly dinner date or a hike with a friend that you've been doing for years. And I truly believe that it's moments like these that can make up the fabric of our life and our wellbeing. Those moments can be dedicated just to you or shared to deepen connections with others.

For me, small rituals that lift my mood and bring me into the now are the groundwork for my overall wellbeing. Little things such as gentle movement, reading a book, arranging flowers, going to the gym or taking time to practise self-massage, are powerful ways to lift my mood and increase my energy.

Self-massage as a self-care ritual

My personal self-massage routines divide into fully conscious rituals and also habits that have become second nature. At first glance, they might appear very similar, as both involve repeated action. But the main difference lies in the level of awareness and intention behind that action.

Every morning and every evening, when applying any of my skincare products, I will undoubtedly massage my face. Without thinking about it too much, maybe even while doing or focusing on something else, I'll perform a series of movements that are by now ingrained in my muscle memory and mind as a habit.

The rituals are where I set the scene, take my time, ask everyone, (including the dog), not to bother me for 10 minutes or more. I might be sitting in bed or on the sofa or behind the bathroom door in front of the mirror. The *where* and *what* might change, but the *how* never does. I might be doing a different massage every time, but I'm always there *for* me, *with* me; present, willing, focused on the action and the way it makes me feel. And that can be addictive.

I don't have a schedule; I try to react to the everyday feedback from my body and mind, choosing the routine that feels right at a particular moment in time. Sometimes, after a long day, I want to sit in bed, covered with a duvet and perform a long, slow scalp massage (*see page 188*). Other times, often before an important meeting or event, I need a pick-me-up, so I turn to my 'special event routine' (*see page 96*).

Self-massage works as a ritual in several ways:

- **The time.** You decide to dedicate five, 10, 15 minutes or more every day to this ritual, putting aside anything that happened before and anything that might happen after. You are here, in the now, present, with nowhere else to be and nothing else to do. That's already meditation.

- **The scene.** Maybe you're alone in the bathroom with soft music playing in the background. Maybe you're sitting on the sofa, covered in blankets, with a scented candle burning. The lights are dimmed and the scene is set. You're already nourishing your senses, bathing your body and mind in an atmosphere that in itself promotes relaxation.

- **The energy.** By taking 10 minutes each day for this practice, you turn off your inner critic and turn on your ability to relax into that part of you that is pure being. Self-massage has the power to stimulate your energy channels, promoting the easy flow of life force through your mind and body, bringing you back into balance and allowing you to face life with inner calm and positivity.

INCORPORATING RITUALS INTO YOUR ROUTINE

If you're still not clear what a ritual is and whether you have one yourself, let me give you some examples:

- **Journalling.** Waking up and dedicating the first five to 10 minutes of your day to putting words down on paper without a specific agenda or questions to answer – just allowing your thoughts and feelings to pour out. Maybe reflecting on the past and planning for the future, but at the same time being in the here and now.

- **Making your morning tea or coffee in a certain way.** A step-by-step process that you religiously adhere to and can't start your day without. A wonderful friend of mine, who's made many trips to Japan and is deeply connected to that culture, has a daily *matcha* ritual. It's a mesmerizing process to watch and even more incredible to be a part of. Slow, intentional, simply beautiful.

- **Taking a walk.** Another good friend of mine, closes his laptop at 2 p.m. every working day of the week, without fail, and goes for a 15-minute walk around a local park. This walk is scheduled in his calendar and the ritual is only cancelled if there's an emergency.

- **A weekly/monthly/yearly catch-up or tradition you've scheduled with your friends or family.** You might not even remember how it started, but you don't remember life before it.

- **Mindful cooking and eating.** This is not a sandwich-on-the-go kind of situation. This is not the time when cooking is seen as a chore. Instead, it's a process that might start with planning: shopping for ingredients, prepping, cooking and assembling the meal. Meals taken either alone or shared can hold a lot of memories for many of us. So maybe, for this ritual, follow your grandma's special recipe that you loved as a child.

- **Meditation or conscious breathing.** Whatever time of the day you choose to do it, consistent mindful practice has been proven to improve many aspects of our lives.

- **Slow, mindful reading.** Focusing on your chosen read brings you to the present moment, calms your breathing (unless you're into thrillers or horror stories!) and offers a welcome escape. Reading widens our horizons and expands our imagination.

- **Face massage.** Turning a daily activity such as washing your face into something more can give you the energy boost or the grounding that you're looking for.

By choosing a ritual or an activity that resonates with you, you create your own emotional and physical transformation, one that will bring positive effects for the mind and spirit and longevity for the body. Now, who doesn't want that?

Weaving the ritual of self-massage into our daily/weekly routines is the maintenance we all need – not a once-a-month pedicure that we think of as a self-care treat, but daily maintenance that sustains our inner calm, physical wellbeing and sharp mind. Dedication to our personal self-care allows us to show up as better individuals in all aspects of our lives, supporting and maintaining the positive, balanced lifestyle we want to commit to in the long term.

Self-massage has other benefits, too, including helping to dispel tension or pain in the body and clearing the mind through the meditative aspect and connection to the breath. We'll explore these and many more benefits in the next chapter.

The Benefits of Face Massage

Self-massage, and specifically face massage, has many undeniable physical benefits, as well as less-visible effects, one of which is its impact on the lymphatic system. Understanding the lymphatic system and where the lymph nodes are allows for better purification of the skin and gives you a good grounding before getting started with the core routines in Part II, so let's dive into that first.

Boosts the Lymphatic System

The lymphatic system is an essential and often under-appreciated component of the circulatory, immune and metabolic systems. It's a network of vessels, nodes and ducts that collect and circulate excess fluid in the body.

The most important functions of the lymphatic system are:

- It maintains the balance of fluids in the body, collecting, purifying and draining excess fluids. This helps to prevent swelling and edema (a build-up of fluid in the body), which can occur after surgery, with a diet high in salt, with prolonged sitting or standing and during pregnancy.

- It supports and facilitates our immune system by producing and releasing lymphocytes (a type of white blood cell) and other immune cells. These cells look for and destroy invaders, such as bacteria, viruses, parasites and fungi, that may enter the body. Think of them as rubbish collectors that filter out bacteria and toxins that can cause disease and inflammation in the body.

- It facilitates dietary fat absorption, as well as fat-soluble vitamins from our intestine that it transports into the bloodstream.

- It maintains a healthy environment in the digestive tract.

- It improves circulation.

- It reduces inflammation. Low-level chronic inflammation has a role to play in almost all illnesses of the Western world. It can also result in infections and autoimmune disorders.

When your lymphatic system is functioning properly, you feel full of energy, clear-headed and ready to take on the world. You sleep well and you digest and eliminate food efficiently. When your system is stagnant, however, you can feel exactly the opposite: you get sick often, need a nap in the afternoon, might get aches and pains you can't explain and can be constipated. So, looking after your lymphatic system is as important as brushing your teeth and having health check-ups.

Your lymphatic system doesn't have a pump (unlike the cardiovascular system that has a heart to pump the blood around), so its flow relies on movement and the contraction of muscles for stimulation – this is where self-massage comes in. By stimulating the flow of lymph around the body with your own two hands, you promote better circulation and the most efficient elimination of your body's waste and toxins. Better circulation also means better delivery of nutrients to cells, providing a boost to your immune system.

A fact that always blows my mind is that one-third of all our lymph nodes are located from the neck up. The head and neck region alone contains more than 300 lymph nodes, which highlights the importance of massaging your neck and face. On page 70 you'll find a full lymphatic drainage routine that you can perform two to three times a week; however, most routines in this book will include moves and exercises designed to stimulate it.

I have no expectation that you should remember the different lymph nodes, but I hope the image on the next page will help you to visualize where they are and give you an idea as to why the routines work on certain areas.

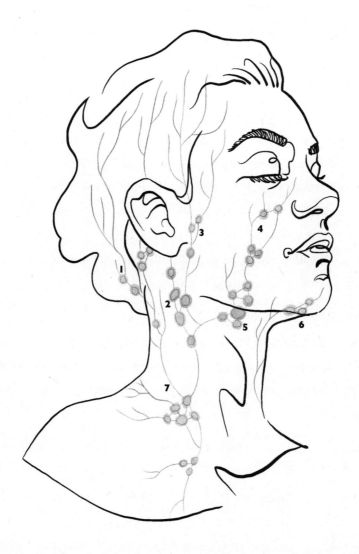

The main lymph nodes: 1. Occipital and posterior auricular **2.** Anterior and posterior cervical **3.** Preauricular **4.** Facial **5.** Submandibular **6.** Submental **7.** Supraclavicular

LYMPHATIC BOOST EXERCISE

I'd love to share with you a practice that boosts your whole body's lymphatic system. This method is designed to stimulate your lymphatic system to promote fluid flow, increase blood flow and nutrient delivery to all the tissues and eliminate waste and toxins from the body. This results in a better functioning lymphatic system, stronger immunity and boosted energy levels. It only takes a few minutes and I'd recommend doing it once a day.

Six points to focus on

1. Collarbone (below and above)
2. Side of the neck
3. Shoulder joint and armpits
4. Abdomen
5. Groin area
6. Behind the knees

How to do it

Tap, rub or massage the above areas to stimulate the nodes, spending 5–10 seconds on each point:

- Start with the collarbone and the side of the neck.
- Move to the shoulder joints and armpits to promote lymph flow.
- Rub and tap your abdomen.
- Find the crease of the groin and tap over it, doing circles over the crease.

- Rub above and below the crease of both knees to stimulate lymph flow.

- Finish with bouncing on your toes for 20 seconds, without taking your feet off the ground.

Once completed, you body will detox, so you might feel slightly nauseous, tired, headachy or dizzy. This is a sign that toxins are moving through your body and going through the process of elimination. Drink plenty of water to aid this process.

Note: Don't try this if you're pregnant, have a heart or circulation disorder, an acute infection or have been diagnosed with cancer.

Plumper, More Nourished Skin

A question I get asked a lot is, 'Won't moving my skin around create more wrinkles?' Let me bust this popular myth right now: face massage can actually improve the overall appearance of skin. Not only can it enhance the overall quality, texture and glow of the skin on your face, neck and chest, but it can also reduce existing lines and slow down the appearance of new ones. To understand how, it's important to know that there are two types of wrinkles:

1. **Dynamic wrinkles:** These develop from repeated facial movements. If you pucker your lips around a straw frequently, for example, you might get lip lines. Or if frowning is your go-to facial expression to show concern, worry or even surprise, then frown lines or 'angry 11s' might become unwelcome guests between your brows.

2. **Static wrinkles:** These result from a loss of elasticity and the takeover of gravity. Jowls, for example, are static.

Dynamic wrinkles can be addressed by releasing tension in the muscles that are overused and by lengthening them. Static wrinkles benefit from massage as it promotes collagen and elastin production, which act as scaffolding and building blocks for your skin, providing support and structure. Whether you're working with existing wrinkles or maybe trying to delay the appearance of new ones, relaxing overactive muscles stops the wrinkles from forming and improves those that have already graced your body. Facial massage has the power to relax the dynamic muscles, so they can't press your skin into new lines.

There are, of course, other factors that contribute to the appearance of lines and wrinkles besides the natural process of ageing and repetitive movements, such as:

• environmental factors including the sun, cold and wind

• poor blood flow

• dehydration and dryness

• poor lymphatic flow

Some of these are difficult to control and to have any effect on or influence over, but some are very much in your hands. Facial massage includes tissue manipulation that increases blood flow, which, in turn, brings fresh nutrients to the skin and oxygenates it. Using the right products also helps with hydration, as dehydration often leads to thinning of the skin and promotes the development of fine lines, wrinkles and crow's feet (*we'll be taking a look at skincare on page 34*).

Lines and wrinkles on your face are the marks of a life lived with laughter and joy – they're a map of your journey through the years. Those repetitive movements I mentioned above can also include smiling, laughing or crying from happiness. And I believe in celebrating these emotions.

The routines, especially those for the target areas in Part IV, will offer you ways to improve lines and wrinkles, but they're also so much more than that. I hope you'll get to experience not just the physical benefits, but also the benefits that go beyond the skin, which we'll look at now.

Counters Harmful Effects of Stress on the Body

To understand how face massage can help you to destress, we first need to explore how stress affects the body. The effects of stress on the whole body are complex and profound, but I've tried to package the extensive information out there into this short, but hopefully comprehensive, section. In my opinion, understanding this is fundamental to driving and motivating us to making positive changes. We'll not only dig into the effects of stress on different body systems, but also explore ways to reduce, manage and eliminate it from our lives.

The word 'stress' immediately sparks a negative emotion in our minds, but stress can be brief, situational and a positive force that can motivate actions and performance. For example, some athletes perform better under pressure. And sometimes with an important meeting or interview ahead, the nervousness we feel can drive us to better preparation that allows us to show up with more confidence on the day. However, frequent, prolonged exposure to stress has a much more profound negative, long-term effect on the body, resulting in problems such as chronic illnesses, diseases and even depression.

There are 11 organ systems in the body and all of them suffer with prolonged exposure to stress. Let's look a little closer at just a few of these now:

- **Musculoskeletal:** Chronic stress causes the muscles in the body to be in a more or less constant state of guardedness and engagement, which can result in muscle pain in the lower back and upper body. Chronic muscle tension can cause tension-type headaches and migraines.

- **Endocrine:** When we're stressed, our adrenal glands produce more cortisol, the so-called stress hormone. While cortisol is essential in stressful situations where we have to act fast, overproduction of this hormone can cause chronic fatigue, metabolic disorders (such as diabetes and obesity) and depression.

- **Cardiovascular:** Constant stress experienced over a prolonged period of time can contribute to long-term problems for our heart and blood vessels. Experiencing a consistent and ongoing increase in heart rate and elevated levels of blood pressure can take a toll on the body. This ongoing stress can increase the risk of hypertension, heart attack or stroke.

- **Respiratory:** Hyperventilation and shortness of breath are common symptoms of stress and can be very uncomfortable. Studies have shown that, in some cases, acute stress can cause asthma attacks.

- **Gastrointestinal:** Our gut has a closer link with our brain than we often assume – think of the expressions 'butterflies in the stomach' and our 'gut feeling.' Stress can affect brain–gut communication and may trigger pain, bloating and other gut discomfort. Stress is associated with changes in gut bacteria that can, in turn, influence mood. It can also affect our hunger, pushing us towards stress-related eating or refusing to eat at all, throwing our wellbeing off balance.

- **Reproductive:** Stress has a direct effect on our sexual desire. It can also impact the production of testosterone and sperm production in males and can cause absent or irregular menstrual cycles, more painful periods and changes to the length of cycles in females.

- **Nervous:** Our autonomic nervous system (ANS) is divided into the sympathetic nervous system (SNS) and the parasympathetic nervous system (PNS). When the body is stressed, the SNS contributes to what's known as the fight-or-flight response, during which the hormones adrenalin and cortisol are released to prepare the body to respond to an emergency situation. When that happens, many systems of the body are affected: our heart rate increases, our pupils dilate and our digestion slows down. Chronic stress results in long-term stimulation of the fight-or-flight response and long-term stress-induced secretion of adrenalin and cortisol is associated with consequences such as high blood glucose levels, which can lead to type 2 diabetes and hypertension (high blood pressure), which, in turn, can lead to cardiovascular disease. The PNS, on the other hand, controls the rest-and-digest response and works to conserve our energy, reduce our heart rate and stimulate our digestive organs. It acts as a brake to our stress when danger is not present. Being in this mode means we are more relaxed and focused.

In addition to the effect of stress on our organ systems, it's also connected to premature ageing. You know those lines between your brows and around your eyes? We call them 'frown lines' and 'angry 11s' for a reason – our emotions are revealed on our skin often without us being aware.

Have you ever heard of psychodermatology? Well, admittedly, neither had I before I started researching for this book. Psychodermatology is a new and emerging subspecialty of both psychiatry and dermatology and addresses the interaction between our mind and skin. As we know, psychiatry focuses on the internal, less-visible state of our body, addressing psychological symptoms and diseases, while dermatology focuses on the external, visible state of our skin. Connecting both gives us a deeper insight into how one affects the other – something that has, unfortunately, been underestimated in the past. Research now shows that psychological stress negatively impacts the homeostasis, in other words, the balance and protective barrier of the skin. And that, in turn, may act as a driver for some inflammatory skin conditions such as dermatitis, psoriasis and premature ageing.

Skin, being the body's largest organ, reflects exactly what is happening under the surface. Whether it's the repetitive movement of a certain muscle caused by emotions, daily stresses causing lines and wrinkles or the quality of the skin being affected by our emotional state, studies have shown that psychological stress negatively impacts skin barrier function, which leads to an increase in inflammation. The production of adrenal hormones triggered by stress, meanwhile, enlarge our oil glands and stimulate oil production, causing acne and breakouts. Stress also slows down wound healing, which includes acne.

The brain–skin connection is a two-way street that can translate psychological stress from the brain onto the skin and vice versa. Think about the last time you experienced stress and suddenly got flushed or noticed a bead of sweat on your forehead. Or how a sudden flare-up of acne affected your mental health. Stressful situations trigger the production of cortisol, which creates inflammation of the skin.

Repeated stress also creates tension in the body – think raised shoulders, tight chest, clenched jaw and frowning of the brows. And this repetitive movement, in turn, results in physical changes, including increased lines and wrinkles, jowls and even grinding the teeth.

Luckily, there are countless techniques and activities – such as breathwork, nature therapy, warm baths or even cuddling a pet (or a human) – that activate the PNS and have been shown to effectively reduce muscle tension and decrease the occurrence of certain stress-related disorders and symptoms. But this is also where practices like self-massage really shine.

BREATHING EXERCISE

One of my go-to breathing techniques is the 4-7-8 breath developed by Dr Andrew Weil, who refers to it as a 'natural tranquilizer for the nervous system'. It's a wonderful tool you can reach for any time you feel stressed, overwhelmed or just need a moment of calm. This technique involves breathing in for four seconds, holding the breath for seven seconds and exhaling for eight seconds. It can help to reduce anxiety and improve sleep quality. Repeat the cycle as many times as you like and feel the benefits.

How Self-Massage Helps Your Nervous System

As we've discovered, the mind-body connection is a two-way relationship where the mind influences the body and the body influences the mind. Physical action has a direct effect on the way we feel.

Skin has a total surface area of around 1.5–2m^2 and represents around 15 per cent of the total weight of the human body. While senses such as hearing, smell and vision allow us to experience and read the world around us from a distance, touch and therefore our skin, provides us with the most direct and the most intimate contact with our surroundings.

Massage uses touch as the main sense of connection to the body. And there's a deep biological connection between our sense of touch and our general wellbeing. We've all felt a boost to our mood after experiencing the touch of a hand from a loved one, a warm hug, a cuddle with a pet or even an encouraging pat on the back.

Since the beginning of time, touch has been a powerful and important way that animals communicate safety to one another, just as we do now to communicate love, compassion, reassurance and support. And so the physical act of touching your own skin has a profound effect on your nervous system.

In 1887, Thomas Stretch Dowse, MD wrote, 'Some physicians suggest that stress may be responsible for 75 per cent of all disease in the Western world, including skin conditions such as psoriasis and eczema, high blood pressure, backache, poor eyesight and depression... the solution is to use massage therapy.'

When you touch something, the receptors on your skin send signals to your brain. These signals then branch out and travel in two directions. One highway leads to your somatosensory cortex, which receives tactile information from the body, including sensations such as touch, pressure, temperature and pain. So it can turn touch into soft, rough, slow, fast, hot or cold sensations.

The other branch is the emotional cortex, the part that connects emotion to touch. When you self-massage, you stimulate pressure receptors deep under the skin and there's a long chain reaction that stimulates the vagus nerve, a key member of the PNS *(see page 25)*, which tells your body to relax and counterbalances the fight-or-flight response. With this kind of stimulation, we promote relaxation in the body, release feel-good hormones such as dopamine and put a brake on the body's stress response.

THE POSITIVE EFFECTS OF SELF-MASSAGE

- It increases circulation to facial tissues, resulting in a brighter, more youthful complexion and healthier skin.

- It reduces anxiety, elevates mood and aids restful sleep by stimulating the vagus nerve and bringing us into the present moment.

- It lowers levels of the stress hormone cortisol by tapping into our PNS, or rest-and-digest state.

- It reduces puffiness and water retention by stimulating circulation and lymphatic drainage.

- It reduces muscle tension in the body through manual softening and lengthening of overused muscles.

- It slows the appearance of new signs of ageing by improving skin elasticity.

- It lowers blood pressure by reducing stress and anxiety.

- It aids digestion and detoxification through lymphatic drainage and improved toxin elimination.

- It promotes respiratory health through calmer, more conscious breathing.

- It instils calm and quietens both the body and mind by bringing us into the now and acts as a meditation.

- It helps us to focus on positive thoughts and actions by rewarding us through acts of self-love and kindness.

Now that you understand the many benefits of self-massage, I invite you to give face massage a go. Start small and allow it to turn into a good habit and then maybe even a ritual, something you look forward to. Schedule it in your diary or send an invite to a friend so you can both do it at the same time in the comfort of your own homes and then share how you feel afterwards.

Give yourself time, commit to it and notice the change. You may wish to track your self-massage journey by taking before and after pictures. This is not only motivating, it's also fascinating to witness the positive transformation.

Absolutely anyone can practise self-massage; whatever gender you identify with, whatever age your passport states, whatever age you are in your mind, it's something that's truly for everyone, everywhere.

In the next section, we'll look at how to get started with face massage and how to choose the products that are right for you, as well as exploring my dos and don'ts of face massage.

Getting Started

My favourite thing about self-massage is that it's incredibly accessible. Clients often ask me what they need to get started and I always answer: All you need is a clean pair of hands and a clean face – your wellbeing is truly at your own fingertips! Using your hands is the best way to connect with your body and discover any tensions or areas that need some extra love. Of course, some people also like to use a massage agent, which we'll explore below. First, though, it's important to understand your individual skin type.

Discover Your Skin Type

Skin-typing is an important piece of the puzzle when it comes to your skin health. It can help when building your skincare routine, your relationship with the sun and even your diet, but it's also important for finding your perfect fit when it comes to an oil or cream for self-massage.

It's worth noting that your skin type can change over time, for a myriad of reasons, including hormonal changes, age, environmental factors and even stress levels, so it's important to stay in tune with your body and observe the changes it goes through as you move through life.

The main criterion that determines your skin type is how much oil your skin naturally produces. To determine yours, try this simple technique:

• Wash your face (with a gentle, non-foaming, mild cleanser), pat it dry with a clean towel and don't apply any other products.

• Wait for 30 minutes, then assess how your skin looks and feels.

Read through the descriptions of the six main skin types below and see which one(s) most closely align to how your skin feels after those 30 minutes have passed.

Normal

Normal is used to describe well-balanced skin, but that's not to say it's perfect. 'Normal' is not a clinical term, but is more just a guide for people to look for the right skincare. Normal skin is skin that's regular in texture, has few to no blemishes, no sensitivity and balanced hydration levels. It has a balance between oil and water, so doesn't feel greasy or dry to the touch.

Dry

Often characterized by flaking, tight, uncomfortable skin that can appear dull and rough in texture, dry skin is prone to showing more lines. Dryness can be caused by different factors, such as harsh products, age, certain medications, medical conditions and the environment.

Oily

Oily skin often appears shiny thanks to excess oil production. It tends to show more in the T-zone (forehead, nose and chin). Pores might appear bigger and overproduction of oil/sebum can lead to acne and blemishes.

Acne-prone

There can often be an overlap between acne-prone and oily skin, but the main symptom is inflammation, which is directly linked to breakout. Skin can often have a rough texture and appear bumpy because of blackheads and/or whiteheads. Overproduction of oil/sebum that leads to frequent breakouts around the face and neck is another characteristic.

Combination

Combination skin might feel dry in some areas and oily in others. Typically, the T-zone is more prone to oiliness, while the cheeks are dry. Seasonal climate changes and genetics both have an effect on combination skin.

Sensitive

Sensitive skin is not skin that might have once had a reaction to a potent product (think an acid toner or a retinol night cream) – that's simply skin that hasn't yet built up tolerance to an active ingredient. Instead, sensitive skin can typically feel itchy, dry and burning. It might have frequent flare-ups due to external factors like hot showers or baths, exercise, food, fragrance or dyes. Sensitive skin can also be a feature of other skin types, so you could have dry and sensitive skin or acne-prone and sensitive skin, for example.

Skincare

Depending on your skin type, there are a few different products you can use for self-massage:

- cleansing balm or oil

- cleansing cream

- facial oil

- face cream

Before we dive into the magic world of creams and oils, my advice is if you're massaging with an oil, wash it off after the routine with your regular cleanser and continue with your normal skincare, applying appropriate serums and moisturizers. This will ensure you're minimizing congestion and maximizing hydration.

K'S TIP

A quick massage while cleansing is one of my favourite ways to consistently include massage into my daily routine. You probably cleanse your face without fail at least once a day anyway, so introducing a few simple moves into your routine will stimulate blood flow and lymphatic drainage and lead to an influx of fresh oxygen and nutrients. It's also a great option for those who are nervous about using oil or who have congestion or acne-prone skin.

Pick a cleanser that gives you a good glide and slide, like a balm or an oil. Perform the cleansing massage below and then wash it off and continue with your normal skincare routine.

You can do this quick cleansing massage morning and evening to release muscle tension, promote blood flow and maximize product efficacy:

1. Apply your product of choice all over your face and neck.

2. Wet your hands thoroughly.

3. Clench your hands into fists and, using your knuckles, massage your neck, cheeks and forehead in circular motions, moving outwards from the centre towards the hairline and ears.

4. Use your index fingers to massage congested areas like sides of the nose, chin and between the brows.

5. Perform circular movements around the eyes, paying extra attention to massaging the brows.

If you've ever felt overwhelmed by the variety of choice in a cosmetics shop – with all the colourful bottles and shiny tubes shouting promises at you from the shelves – then welcome to the club. The beauty market is the most saturated it's ever been and is growing at an alarming rate, so knowing where to start when building your skincare routine can feel like a minefield. My tip is – start simple. Think about the three main pillars: cleansing, hydration and protection. Once you cover those three, you can start adding actives that target different concerns that can change with age, the seasons and hormonal variables.

1. **Cleansing:** A very important part of your routine, this helps to remove dead skin cells, dirt, excess oil, product, sweat and dust. If your skin isn't cleansed properly, dirt and pollution accumulate at the surface of your skin and could potentially contribute to breakouts, dehydration and premature ageing. Our skin also has its own microbiome, so countless bacteria populate the surface of our skin. But not all bacteria are bad! Some help to maintain the homeostasis, or balance, of our skin and strengthen our skin barrier. So choose a non-stripping, gentle cleanser that doesn't leave your skin feeling tight or dry.

2. **Hydration:** This is the next essential step to healthy skin. And healthy skin is beautiful skin. Your skin comes with a natural protective barrier that guards it against external damage, such as environmental pollution, oxidation from UV rays, weather changes and more.

Moisturizers can provide hydration and other benefits that protect and even strengthen that barrier. They're normally formulated with oils, water, humectants, emollients and other agents that soften, hydrate and balance your skin.

You can choose a cream, gel or lotion for your moisturizer, depending on your skin type, and apply twice a day as a rule of thumb, morning and evening. There's no one-size-fits-all, so having a consultation with a dermatologist will help you determine your skin type and pick the right product for you.

3. **Protection:** The final step in your morning routine. And we're talking about SPF here, which stands for sun protection factor. Wearing sunscreen year-round will prevent skin damage from UV rays and minimize your risk of skin cancers and premature ageing.

    Look for a broad-spectrum formula, which means it protects against both UVB and UVA rays; if the product isn't labelled as broad-spectrum, it only protects against UVB. UVB causes burning of the skin, while UVA causes photoageing, such as wrinkles or loss of collagen, and promotes the formation of brown spots on the skin. As a general rule, SPF 30 is the minimum I'd advise to use all year round and, when applying, use the length of two fingers (the first and the middle) for the face and neck.

K'S TIP

Skincare needn't be expensive. There are so many changes we can make to our daily routines that will help transform our skin and they're completely free! Here are three of my favourite cost-free skincare tips:

1. Clean your makeup brushes. These must be cleaned every seven to 10 days as brushes allow bacteria to breed and thrive, which can cause inflammatory skin conditions and acne.

2. Avoid face cloths. Face cloths are another breeding ground for bacteria (especially as they stay so damp). If you like to use them, make sure you use a clean one each time. Muslin cloths can be washed and dried much more quickly than standard cloths.

3. Wash your pillowcases. They need to be washed more often than you might think – we spend so much time lying on them. Silk pillowcases are kinder on our skin and hair, so consider swapping your current cases for silk ones if you're able to.

Choosing the Right Oil or Cream for Your Massage

Oils

If you have oily or acne-prone skin, you might get goosebumps (and not the good kind) when you hear the word 'oil' when it comes to skincare. Oils certainly have a controversial reputation, but I'm here to tell you that, regardless of your skin type, you can and even should be introducing one into your routine. There are countless potential benefits you might be missing out on if you don't.

Plant-based oils are rich in antioxidants and essential fatty acids, as well as vitamins that help strengthen our skin barrier and nourish and improve skin elasticity. Regardless of your skin type, essential fatty acids are as important for skin health as they are in your diet. Topical application of skincare with fatty acids helps with protection from UV radiation and sunburn – a critical step to prevent premature skin ageing and wrinkles. But the wrong oil can cause pore clogging, which can lead to inflammation and acne. So the goal is to avoid or decrease the use of oils that are 'comedogenic', which clog pores and may cause breakouts.

With an overwhelming, and even confusing, choice of facial oils, it can be hard to know how to pick the one that's right for you. I hope the guidance here will make it a little easier. First, we need to look at something called a 'comedogenic rating'. This is a scale that shows how likely a specific ingredient is to clog your pores. The scale ranges from 0 to 5, with 0 being non-comedogenic and 5 being the most severely comedogenic:

- 0 – non-comedogenic (does not clog pores)
- 1 – slightly comedogenic (very low chance of clogging pores)
- 2 – moderately low comedogenic (may clog pores for some, but be fine for most)
- 3 – moderately comedogenic (will clog acne-prone/oily skin types)

- 4 – fairly high comedogenic (will clog pores for almost all skin types)

- 5 – highly comedogenic (will clog pores)

The table opposite displays the comedogenic rating for different oils. The ratings listed here have been derived and compiled from various sources.

In summary, the oils I'd mostly avoid on the face include:

- coconut oil

- flaxseed oil

- palm oil

- soybean oil

In addition, other oils that are higher in oleic acid, like cocoa and shea butter, might also encourage breakouts in those who are prone.

Of course, if you've been using the oils mentioned above and your skin feels nourished, balanced and mostly clear, then you've made the right choice for you. Skin, like anything else, is personal. There are no universal recommendations, so always try a new product on a small area of facial skin first. If you're not sure or have a concern, I'd advise consulting a dermatologist.

On page 42, I've included a round-up of my favourite oils.

NAME	COMEDOGENIC RATING	SKIN TYPE(S)	COMPOSITION
Almond oil	2	Dry, sensitive, acne-prone	High in oleic acid
Argan oil	0	Most skin types	High in oleic acid and linoleic acid
Avocado oil	3	Dry, acne-prone	High in oleic acid
Cocoa butter	4	Ideal for body/eye area, not for oily/acne-prone	High in oleic and stearic acid
Coconut oil	4	Very dry, best for body use	High in lauric acid
Grapeseed oil	1	Most skin types	High in linoleic acid
Hempseed oil	0	Most skin types, incl oily/acne-prone	High in linoleic acid, moderate in linolenic acid
Jojoba oil	2	Most skin types, incl oily/acne-prone	High in eicosenoic acid
Rosehip oil	1	Oily/acne-prone	High in linoleic acid, moderate in linolenic acid
Squalane oil	0-1	Most skin types	High in omega-2

My Go-To Oils

Squalane

This has been a personal go-to for many years and is a great place to start if you're wary of or new to facial oils. Squalane oil, not to be confused with 'squalene,' which is naturally produced by the body, is a fascinating ingredient as it works very much like the skin's own oil to prevent moisture loss. The skin, therefore, instantly recognizes squalane and knows how to use it. Besides being a great moisturizing agent, squalane works with other antioxidants and helps to protect against UV damage.

Great for: most skin types

Rosehip oil

Rosehip is a beautiful, nourishing oil that has anti-inflammatory properties. Because of its high concentrations of vitamins A, B and E, rosehip oil is known for its exceptional regenerative and healing properties. It also contains vitamin C, which can help reduce the appearance of fine lines and wrinkles, brighten the skin and help fight free radicals in the skin.

Great for: acne-prone, oily or combination skin

Hempseed oil

This is a non-comedogenic oil that helps to hydrate without causing blackheads or breakouts. It's also rich in linolenic acid, which makes the oil effective at reducing inflammation and encouraging skin regeneration.

Great for: oily or acne-prone skin

Grapeseed oil

Grapeseed oil is a lightweight oil that's known for its antimicrobial and anti-inflammatory properties. It also contains high levels of omega-6 fatty acids and vitamin E. Rich in polyphenol, grapeseed oil is packed with antioxidants that can help reduce the signs of ageing, such as pigmentation, fine lines and wrinkles.

Great for: normal, oily, sensitive or combination skin

Jojoba oil

Want to know a fun fact? Jojoba oil isn't actually an oil – it's a wax ester and is composed almost entirely (about 97 per cent) of monoesters of long-chain fatty acids (wax ester) and alcohols. Human sebum also contains wax esters, which means that jojoba oil is very close to our skin's natural oil. It hydrates, offers antioxidant protection and soothes without clogging the skin.

Great for: normal, oily and combination skin

Creams

Cream would be my second or even third choice as a massage agent, as most moisturizers have a higher concentration of water compared to oils and cleansing oils/balms, which leads to quicker evaporation and absorption. But if that's all you have or is what you prefer, then I support anything that facilitates your journey of being consistent with facial massage and allows you to enjoy the process.

Choose a simple moisturizer without actives (like retinoids or acids) that has a nice slip to it. If, as soon as you apply a moisturizer, your skin absorbs it and feels dry to the touch, it's time to step up your hydration and treat yourself to a richer, better-performing product.

K'S TIP

Your hands are magic and are all you really need to practise self-massage. But if you're interested in expanding your routines, then *gua sha* is a wonderful ancient healing technique that you can introduce as well. *Gua sha* is a beauty ritual that uses a tool to stimulate blood and lymph flow, as well as release tension in your muscles without too much pressure on your wrists and hands. It also provides a very even pressure on the skin and covers a larger area, compared to your hands. Your tool can be made of any material: jade, rose quartz, bian stone or metal.

When using your *gua sha* tool, make sure to keep a few things in mind:

- Ensure that your *gua sha* tool, hands and face are clean.

- Apply oil or cream for the massage so as not to drag the skin.

- Hold your tool almost flat against your skin or at a 30-degree angle.

- Clean your *gua sha* tool with warm soapy water after every use.

- Breathe!

My favourite way to use a *gua sha* tool is to place it in warm water for five minutes before use for an added soothing, releasing effect. It's a wonderful way to unwind before bed or during the day. Focus on areas of tension like the chest, neck, back of the shoulders, jaw, forehead and temples. Re-submerge and heat up your tool as many times as you need.

Getting to Know the Facial Muscles

Now, you might wonder why you need to know about the muscles in the face and I promise that I'm not going to get too technical here, but having some understanding of the facial muscles and their location means you'll know which ones to concentrate on for tension release and addressing any areas of concern. It also helps you to understand which direction to move your fingers in and which areas of the face and neck to focus on.

There are approximately 43 muscles in the face and 20 in the neck, which allow us to make countless expressions from sadness and surprise to joy. Many anatomists and studies estimate that we use between 12 and 17 muscles just to smile alone. If you think about all the repetitive movements that happen in our face, every one of them triggers certain muscles to contract and shorten, which changes the shape of our face and sometimes creates creases and folds. With massage, we want to work on those hard-working muscles to relax and lengthen them and, in turn, allow the skin to come back to its resting, smooth position after every one of those contractions.

You may want to approach the next bit of information sitting in front of a mirror. Read out loud the name of the muscle (you can add an accent – I quite like Italian) and then try to activate it. Even if you can't quite get it to move, I hope you have fun in the process. You can refer to the image on page 49 for some visual help.

- **Buccinator:** Compresses the cheeks and expels air between the lips (think of playing the flute). Massaging this muscle helps to release tension in the jaw and improve nasolabial folds.

- **Corrugator supercilii:** Draws the eyebrows down and in, as in frowning. Working with this muscle can improve frown lines and reduce tension between the brows.

- **Depressor anguli oris:** Pulls the corners of the mouth downwards, creating a sad mouth look. When toning this muscle, we can improve jowls, lift the corners of the mouth and even reduce a double chin.

- **Depressor labii inferioris:** Pulls the lower lip downwards and a little to one side. Massaging this muscle helps to improve the jawline, a double chin and mouth lines.

- **Levator labii superioris:** Raises the upper lip, exposing the upper teeth and opens the nostrils. Massaging this muscle helps to improve nasolabial folds and mouth lines.

- **Masseter:** Responsible for the elevation, and some protraction, of the lower jaw. Working with this muscle helps to relieve tension in the jaw and head and relieve temporomandibular (TMJ) disorder.

- **Mentalis:** Raises and protrudes the lower lip, causing the chin to wrinkle. Working in this area helps to smooth the chin and sculpt the jawline.

- **Occipitofrontalis:** Raises the eyebrows and causes the forehead to wrinkle. Working with this muscle helps to improve forehead lines and release tension headaches.

- **Orbicularis oculi:** Closes the eyelids and tightens the skin of the forehead. Working with this circular muscle helps to improve crow's feet and fine lines around the eyes and de-puff the area.

- **Orbicularis oris:** Closes the mouth and compresses, puckers and wrinkles the lips. Working with this muscle helps to release tension around the mouth, improve lip lines and wrinkles, lift the corners of the mouth and plump the lips.

- **Platysma:** Depresses the lower jaw and lip, draws the angle of the mouth downwards and tightens and wrinkles the skin of the neck. Working with this muscle helps to improve our posture, minimize lines on the neck and improve a double chin and jowls.

- **Procerus:** Wrinkles the skin across the bridge of the nose and pulls the eyebrows downwards. Working with this muscle helps to improve angry 11s.

- **Risorius:** Pulls the angle of the mouth out and back, as in smiling. Working with this muscle helps to improve the lines around the mouth as well as improve jowls and the oval of the face.

- **Temporalis:** Helps your jaw to close. Working with this large muscle helps to improve the whole oval of the face, as well as release tension in the temples and head.

- **Zygomaticus:** Raises the lip, helping to create a smile or laugh. Tension in this muscle is often responsible for our nasolabial folds, so working with it helps to reduce them.

I love this exercise as it creates a deeper connection and understanding between the mind and body. I really wish the teachers at my school had implemented this approach – I might have learned more then!

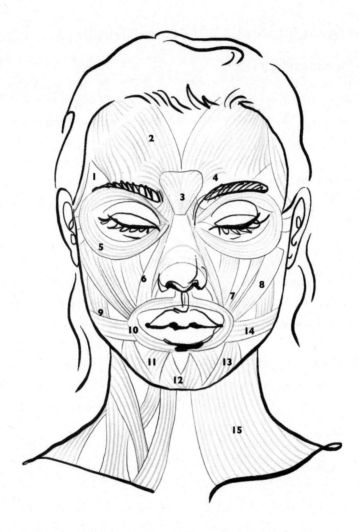

Discovering the muscles of the face: 1. *Temporalis* **2**. *Occipitofrontalis* **3.** *Procerus* **4**. *Corrugator supercilii* **5**. *Orbicularis oculi* **6**. *Levator labii superioris* **7**. *Buccinator* **8**. *Zygomaticus* **9**. *Masseter* **10**. *Orbicularis oris* **11.** *Depressor labii inferioris* **12.** *Mentalis* **13**. *Depressor anguli oris* **14.** *Risorius* **15.** *Platysma*

The Dos and Don'ts of Face Massage

My face massage Dos...

- **Cleanse your face and hands** before you begin to create a clean slate, free from harmful bacteria that can cause inflammation in the skin. Use gentle cleansers on the face to avoid dryness.

- **Wash your face after the massage**. This isn't a must but is the safest option to avoid congestion and breakouts. Skin and its reaction to different products is very individual. However, it's important to remember that massage stimulates the tissues and softens the skin, so my advice is always either to massage with a cleansing balm or oil that then gets washed off, or with an oil that you can cleanse off and then continue with your normal skincare routine.

- **Practise anywhere, anytime**. I'm a great believer in routine, but it can definitely be easier said than done. So, whether you can commit to one minute or 10, dedicate that time to you. I sometimes find myself on a London tube or bus, massaging my forehead or sitting with my eyes closed – but beneath my eyelids I'm practising eye yoga *(see page 195)*, so use whatever free time you have and you'll soon see the benefits.

- **Breathe**. Your breath is the only system in the body you have direct control over – and it's powerful. Holding your breath can create unnecessary tension in the body and the aim of the self-massage routines is to tap into a calmer nervous system and reduce stress.

So, while you practise your routines, try to stay aware of a calm, consistent, mindful breath, inhaling through the nose and exhaling through the mouth, unless otherwise specified.

- **Set the scene.** If you have some time and space, especially for the nighttime routine on page 80, create an atmosphere that entices you to practise – use candles, incense, dimmed lights, your favourite music, blankets or whatever creates a peaceful, soothing atmosphere for you. And if you're looking to raise your vibrations, then maybe it's a case of 'Dancing Queen' or your favourite up-beat song playing through your speaker while you go through your morning routine (*see page 75*).

- **Use a mirror.** If you're new to facial massage, a mirror will be your best ally. Go slow, take your time and observe your reflection in the mirror. While practising, ask yourself these questions: Are my shoulders lifted and tense? Am I unintentionally wrinkling my forehead while working on my jawline? Are my hands moving evenly and symmetrically on both sides? Watch, adjust and continue.

- **Take pictures.** Tracking your progress and seeing the results can really make a difference to your motivation and validate your dedication to the practice.

- **Follow the massage lines.** I've created an image on the next page that you can always refer back to.

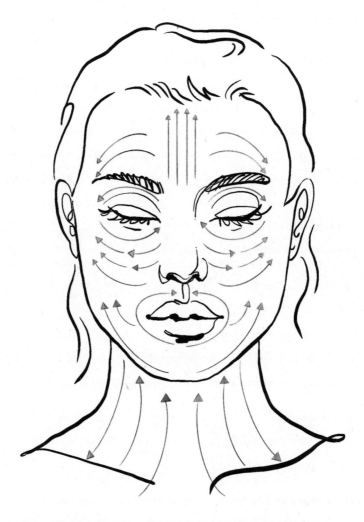

The massage lines to follow when performing exercises

My face massage Don'ts...

- **Don't massage over active acne**. If you have whiteheads, sore bumps or inflammation on the skin, then it's best to avoid massaging over and close to that area. Knocking a spot can cause bleeding that might allow the spread of bacteria, which will slow down healing and can cause scarring. You can, however, practise a gentle lymphatic drainage massage to promote blood flow and toxin elimination (*see page 70*). If your skin is healing, focus on your neck and chest.

- **Don't forget to wash your hands and face before the massage**. Spreading bacteria on your face can cause breakouts and acne.

- **Don't apply hard pressure.** You should never feel pain when practising facial massage. Some areas of tension might feel uncomfortable at first, but go slowly and check in with yourself for what feels right for you.

- **Don't skip the warm-up sequence** (*see page 61*).

- **Don't use unsuitable creams or serums for massage**. The role of a massage agent is to lubricate and to ensure that your fingers and hands glide over the skin. If you're using a water-based product that quickly absorbs into the skin, the chances are you'll end up dragging and creasing the tissues or reapplying too many times and overfeeding the skin with the ingredients in the chosen product. I'd recommend finding an oil-based product that will give you more glide (*see page 42 for my advice on the best products to use for face massage*).

- **Don't massage while using prescription retinols or taking oral acne medication**, such as Roaccutane (isotretinoin capsules). Some medications or topical prescription creams cause sensitivity and thinning of the skin, so be sure to consult your doctor before practising massage.

Your Questions Answered

Q. How often should I massage my face and how long for?

A. When it comes to how often and how long you should massage your face for, every routine in this book has a specified time and repetition for the exercises, to make it super-easy to incorporate into your day. Of course, practising consistently three to four times a week will give you long-lasting visible and invisible (think calmer, happier self) results, but over the years, I've found that doing something every day for five minutes is more likely to result in sustainable change than practising something once a week for 30 minutes. So, if you're short of time and you just have one minute in the morning while doing your skincare routine, implement a few of your favourite moves from the routines into the product application. This is the easiest way to create a consistent facial massage practice.

Clients often ask me when is the best time to do face massage and my answer is always the same: anytime you have the time. Sometimes putting specific boundaries and expectations on a task can make it less achievable. Many of us lead busy lives; plans can change daily and that's okay!

Got five minutes in the morning? Try the energizing routine (see *page 90*). Got a little longer in the evening and feel like taking your time? The relaxing routine (see *page 86*) would be my go-to.

Just find a moment and space that you can devote to yourself and enjoy.

Q. When will I see results?

A. This will vary considerably from person to person. Things like physical activity, work load, home environment, diet and stress levels all have a role to play in how we look and feel. Acknowledging and taking ownership of this without judgement is important as we're all in different stages of our wellness journey – and every step of it is beautiful.

Some of the exercises and routines might give you immediate results, while some areas require a little more persuasion. Try to focus on and enjoy the process and, when results are revealed, celebrate yourself exactly as you are.

Q. I want to start self-massage but I feel a little overwhelmed.

A. First of all, I get it! You're not alone. Second, you've already made a move in the right direction by reading this book. Did you know that contemplation is the second stage of the Transtheoretical Model (TTM) of health behaviour change? This means you're already further on the path to change than you might have thought. My advice is to start small.

Implementing just one minute of self-massage into your day is already a start, and the way it makes you feel can be contagious. The reflection you see in the mirror, the elevated mood and the lightness you feel in your body are addictive and your habits will form quickly.

Unlike many other self-care practices, self-massage requires only two ingredients: your own magic hands and, if you choose to use one, a massage agent (such as an oil). Start with the warm-up routine on page 61, then try implementing a morning or nighttime routine (*see pages 75 and 80*) and watch it become your go-to moment of self-love.

If you still feel a little daunted, habit stacking can help building a new habit feel more achievable (*see page 58*).

Q. Is it too late to start self-massage if I'm over 50?

A. It's never too late when it comes to self-care and dedicating time to your health and wellness. There's no better day than today to start making small or big changes for the better. All ages can benefit from face massage; you might just have different goals at 20 and 55. Nourishing yourself from the inside and out is ageless.

Q. Can I do face massage if I've had Botox or fillers?

A. It's always important to consult your aesthetician or practitioner about post-treatment care. To avoid displacing Botox to unwanted locations, wait one to two weeks before massaging your face. You can, however, still practise neck and shoulder massages, as well as a gentle lymphatic drainage massage. I would advise not massaging your face after having fillers for at least four to six weeks.

THE POWER OF HABIT STACKING

Habit stacking works by linking a new action or habit to an already existing one so that the two become intertwined in your brain. So, if you want to incorporate face massage as a regular practice into your day, but are feeling a little overwhelmed and don't know where to start, begin by identifying something that's already a habit, that doesn't take a lot of conscious effort, and then add one of the face massage routines from Part II on to it. For example, when applying your face cream or cleansing your face, add a couple of massage moves to that practice every day and soon they'll become intuitive and natural. Alternatively, when you're brushing your teeth, why not try some eye yoga (*see page 195*)?

Habit stacking provides you with a built-in mental reminder to associate one activity with the other.

PART II
THE BASIC ROUTINES

The following pages offer you a library of routines that you can use on a daily basis. I hope some of them will become your go-tos when it comes to taking a moment for yourself.

Please note, before getting stuck into these routines, it's essential that you start with the warm-up sequence (*opposite*) as it warms up the muscles and lymph nodes and allows for a better flow and longer-lasting results.

Warm-Up Sequence

This sequence is designed to warm up the muscles and lymphatic system to maximize the effect of any of the routines that follow. It can also be done as a stand-alone relaxing, releasing practice and helps to release muscle tension that can cause lines and wrinkles. You do not need any oil or product for this massage, just clean hands.

Products: clean skin, no product

Time: 5 minutes

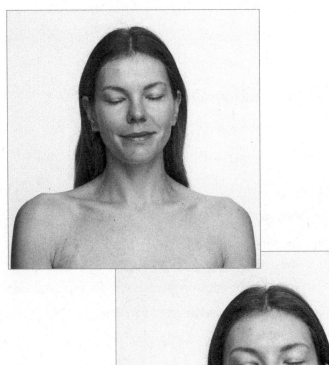

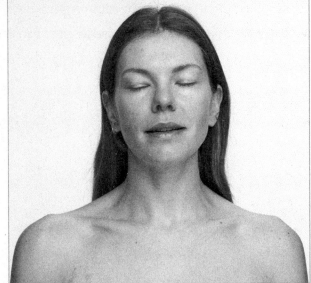

1. Sitting or standing tall, with your spine long, close your eyes and take three deep breaths, breathing in through the nose and sighing out of the mouth with a 'Ha' sound. Let go of any tension with every exhalation.

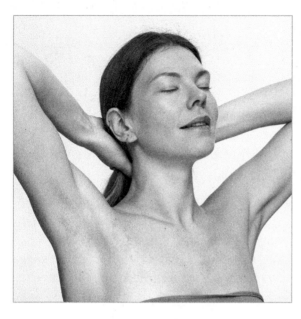

2. Interlace your palms behind your head. As you inhale, open your elbows wide and push your heart and chest forwards.

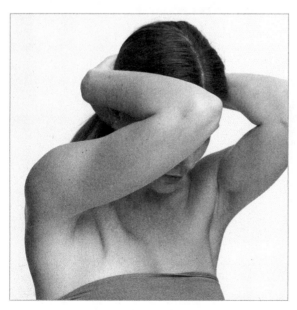

3. As your exhale, tuck in your chin and gently round through your upper back, allowing your elbows to move forwards towards each other. Repeat five times.

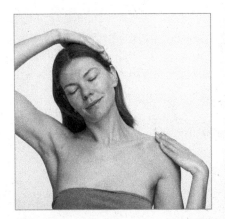 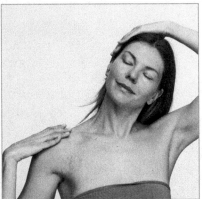

4. Rest one hand over your head and place the other on top of your shoulder. Gently drop your head to the side and stretch your palms away from each other. Hold for two full, deep breaths, switch sides and repeat.

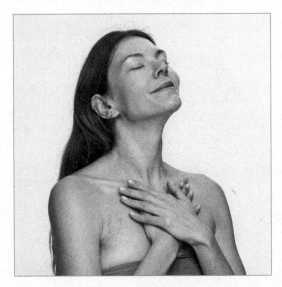

5. Place your palms one on top of the other in the middle of your chest. Relax your shoulders and gently stretch your chin up to the sky. Hold for five seconds. Repeat three times.

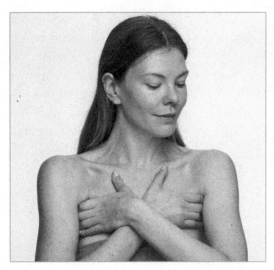

6. Cross your wrists and place your fingertips under your armpits. Gently press into this space three times.

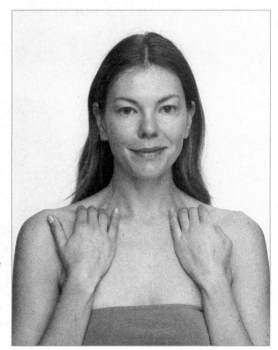

7. Place the fingers of both hands above each collarbone and press lightly three times into the hollow space.

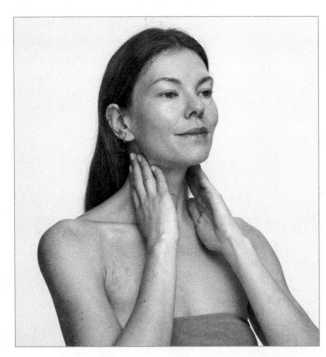

8. With your fingertips on either side of your neck, press lightly in the space below the ears three times and circle three times.

9. With your middle fingers in front and your thumb and index fingers behind your ears, move your hands up and down creating a rubbing motion around the ears. Repeat three times.

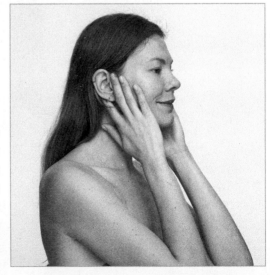

Beginner's Routine

If you're new to facial massage, this is a wonderful place to start and get familiar with the directions of movements and areas to focus on. Refer back to the image on page 52 showing the massage lines if you need to. This is a quick routine you can do every day to give your skin a little boost.

Products: cleanser, cream or oil (see *page 38 for advice on the best products for massage*)

Time: 5–8 minutes

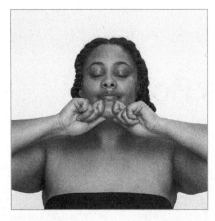

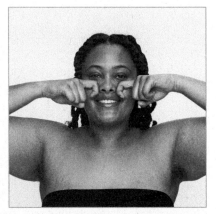

1. Jawline hook: Curl your fingers in. Place your thumbs under your chin, pressing your first fingers to your jawline. Slide out from your chin towards your ears. Repeat five times.

2. Cheek hook: Keeping your index fingers curled, place them on either side of your nose. Slide your fingers out towards your ears. Repeat five times.

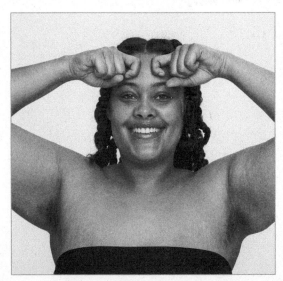

3. Forehead hook: Place your curled index fingers in the middle of your forehead and then slide them out towards your temples. Repeat five times.

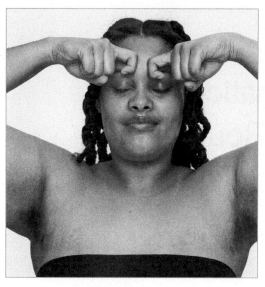

4. Brow hook: Place your curled index fingers between your brows and then slide them out towards your temples. Repeat five times.

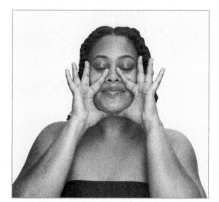

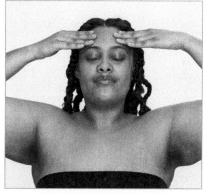

5. Butterfly: With your thumbs under your chin, frame your mouth and nose with your index fingers, opening out your palms. Slide your hands to the sides of your face, gently pressing your index fingers onto your face. Repeat five times.

6. Forehead glide: Place your fingers flat in the middle of your forehead, then gently slide them out towards your temples. Keep your shoulders down and breathe calmly. Repeat five times.

Lymphatic Drainage Routine

This is a personal favourite of mine owing to its overall health and full-body benefits, including:

- the elimination of waste and toxins from the body

- a boost for your immune system

- decreased water retention and heaviness in the limbs

- brighter, healthier skin

This gentle form of massage stimulates the flow of lymphatic fluids in the body and reduces inflammation, which is a cause of ageing and most skin concerns. This massage is done on dry, clean skin, using gentle pressure without dragging the skin. You can do one side first and then the other or both at the same time.

Products: clean skin, no product

Time: 5 minutes

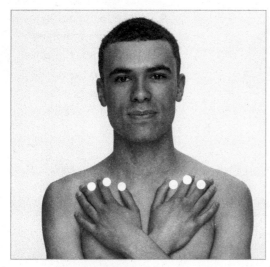

1. Place your fingers above your collarbone. Gently press down and create a circular movement five times. Use opposite hands for each side (right hand on left collarbone, left hand on right collarbone).

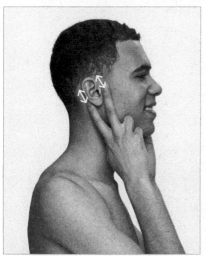

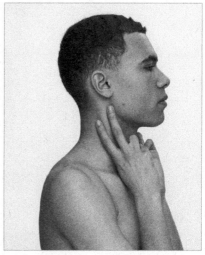

2. Place your index fingers behind your ears and middle fingers in front. Gently press up and down and create a rubbing movement. Repeat five times.

3. Keep your hands in the previous position and sweep them down towards your collarbone. Repeat five times.

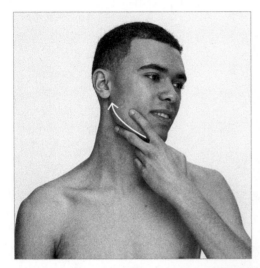

4. Make the peace sign with your first two fingers and sweep them outwards from your chin to your ear five times. Use opposite hands for each side.

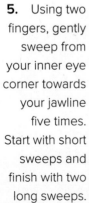

5. Using two fingers, gently sweep from your inner eye corner towards your jawline five times. Start with short sweeps and finish with two long sweeps.

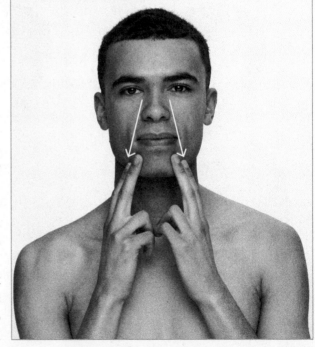

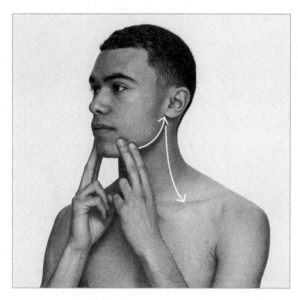

6. Sweep along your jawline, from your chin to your ear and down to your collarbone.

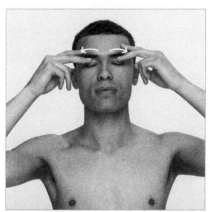

7. Place one finger above and one finger below each eyebrow. Gently sweep out towards your temple five times.

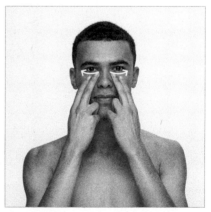

8. Place two fingers into the inner corner of your eyes and sweep under the eye towards your temple five times. Finish with a sweep from your temple to your collarbone.

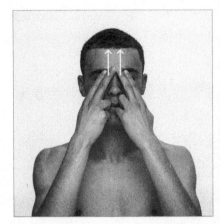

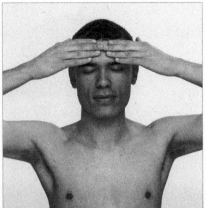

9. Using two fingers on each hand, sweep from the bridge of your nose up towards your hairline 10 times.

10. Using both hands, sweep from the centre of your forehead out towards your temple 10 times.

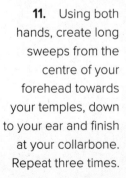

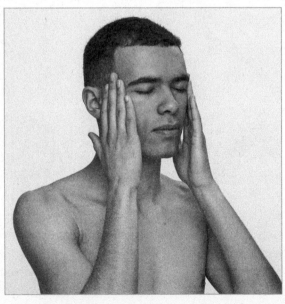

11. Using both hands, create long sweeps from the centre of your forehead towards your temples, down to your ear and finish at your collarbone. Repeat three times.

Morning Routine

This uplifting, de-puffing and awakening routine will set you up for the day. It's my favourite way to start the day, as it boosts your lymphatic and blood flow. Here, we're working to reduce water retention, dark circles and puffiness and revitalize any dullness of the skin. This routine can be performed daily.

Products: cleanser, day cream and eye cream, if using

Time: 5–8 minutes

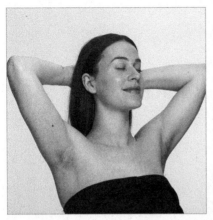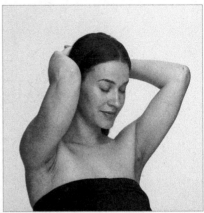

1. Standing cat-cow: Interlace your fingers behind your head. As you inhale, open your elbows wide and push your heart and chest forwards. As you exhale, tuck in your chin and gently round through your upper back, allowing your elbows to come forwards, towards each other. Repeat three times.

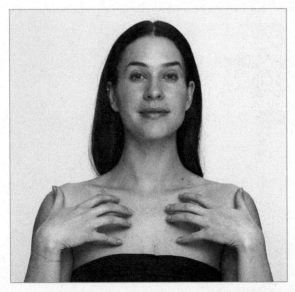

2. Tapping: Using your fingertips, gently tap across your chest and the sides of your neck for 10 seconds.

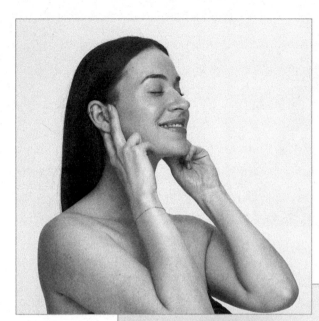

3. Peace fingers: Place your index fingers behind your ears and your middle fingers in front of your ears. Gently press up and down and create a rubbing movement. Repeat five times.

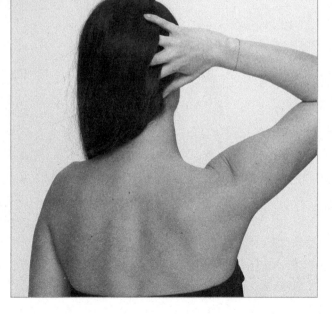

4. Scalp massage: Using your fingers and palms, massage all across the back of your head in circular motions.

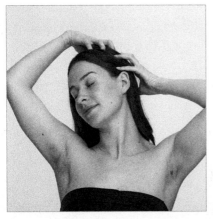

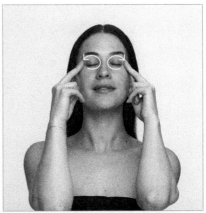

5. Head massage: Using the fingers on both hands, massage your scalp in circular and zig-zag motions all over your head.

6. Eye circles: If using eye cream, apply it with this step. Using your index and middle fingers, gently sweep from the inner corners of your eyes outwards and over the brows. Repeat five times.

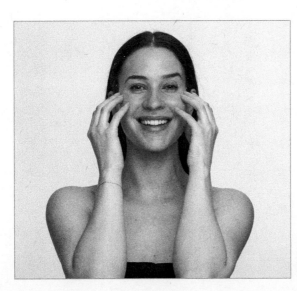

7. Eye tapping: Using your fingertips, gently pat under your eyes, moving from the inner corner outwards. Repeat three times.

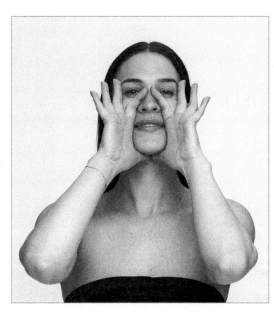

8. Butterfly: If you were using a cleanser before, wash it off now and use this move to apply your face cream. With your thumbs under your chin, frame your mouth and nose with your index fingers, opening out your palms. Slide your hands towards the sides of your face, gently pressing your index fingers onto your face. Repeat three times.

9. Jaw release: Place your knuckles parallel to your jawline under your cheekbones. Slightly open your mouth and massage up and down, pressing the knuckles into the chewing (masseter) muscles for 10 seconds (*see the image on page 49 for reference*). Keep your shoulders relaxed.

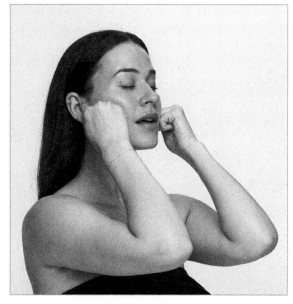

Nighttime Routine

Self-massage helps to relax the body and the mind, softens tension in our muscles and allows us to decompress before bed. This soothing routine taps into your rest-and-digest parasympathetic nervous system (or PNS; *see page 25*) and prepares your body and mind for the best night's sleep. The release of tension in the shoulders, neck and face sheds the stresses of the day and clears the head.

Products: oil or cream

Time: 10–15 minutes

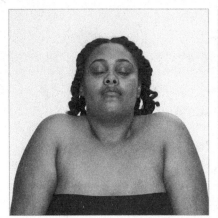 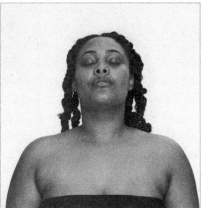

1. Shoulder drop: Inhale and pull your shoulders up towards your ears. As you exhale, sharply drop your shoulders down. Repeat three times.

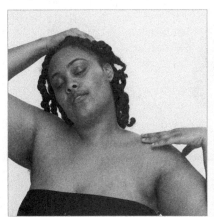 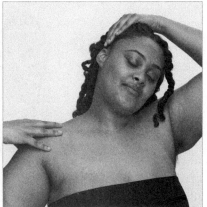

2. Side neck stretch: Dropping your head to one side, gently stretch your head away from your shoulder. Hold for 10 seconds and repeat on the other side.

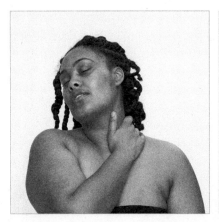
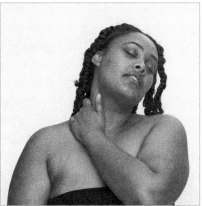

3. Neck massage: Using your opposite hand, massage the side of your neck and the top of your shoulder with your palm for 20 seconds. Repeat on the other side.

4. Jaw release: Place your middle finger on top of your index finger and using your thumb, too, 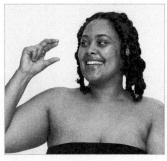 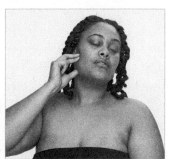 create a 'C' shape. Placing your thumbs under your jawline, press your index and middle fingers into your chewing (masseter) muscle (*see the image on page 49 for reference*), creating a circular movement. Work your way along the whole muscle, feeling for areas of tension.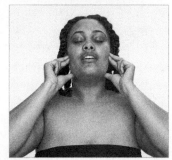

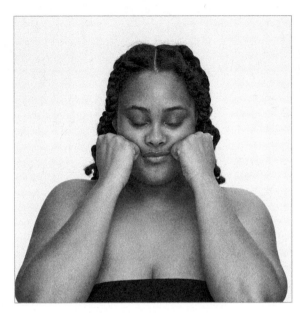

5. Cheekbone release: Create fists and place your knuckles under your cheekbones. Lean your head forwards and hold for 10 seconds. Repeat three times.

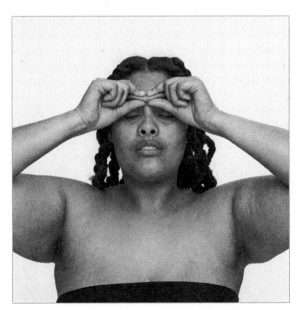

6. Angry 11s pinch: Use your thumbs and index fingers to pinch the space between your brows, creating a fold. Try to grab on to the deeper muscle and not just the skin, to form a fold of about ⅛ inch (4mm). Hold for five seconds while breathing deeply. Repeat three times.

7. Eye circles: Using your ring (or ring and middle) fingers, massage in gentle circles around your eyes. Repeat five times.

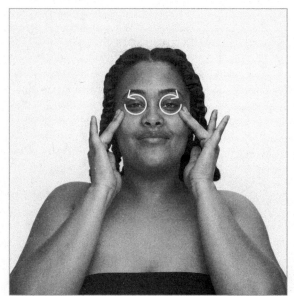

8. Forehead circles: Using your ring and middle fingers, massage in circles moving outwards from the centre of your forehead towards your temples. Repeat twice across your whole forehead.

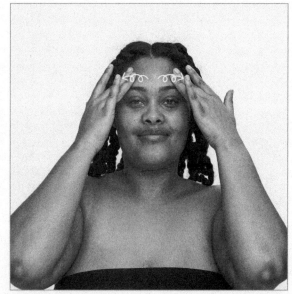

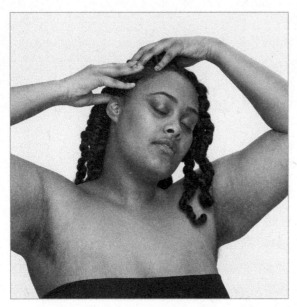

9. Scalp massage: Using your fingertips, massage your scalp across your whole head. Keep your shoulders down and breathe calmly.

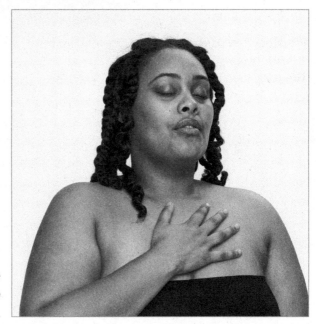

10. End with the 4-7-8 breath (*see page 27*).

Relaxing Routine

This is a lovely routine to help you release and let go, focusing on softening muscle tightness, slowing down the breath and letting go of any tension. We focus on common tension offenders – neck, shoulders, forehead and temples. Move slowly, taking your time. This routine is a fantastic tool at any time of the day to slow things down.

Products: cleanser, facial oil or cream

Time: 10–15 minutes

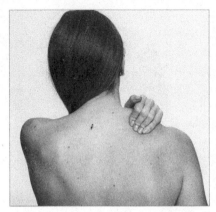 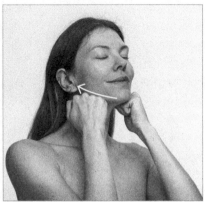

1. Trapezius grab: Place your left palm on top of your right shoulder. Grab onto the muscle and pull it forwards, sliding your fingers towards your collarbone. Repeat five times on each side.

2. Jawline release: Create fists with your hands and place the flat part of your knuckles under your jawline in the centre. Slide out towards your ears and down to your collarbones. Repeat five times.

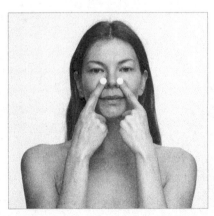 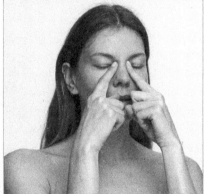

3. Mouth release: Using your index fingers, massage the space on the outside of your nostrils in a circular motion. Repeat five times.

4. Eye tension release: Using your index fingers, massage the inner corners of your eyes in a circular motion. Repeat five times.

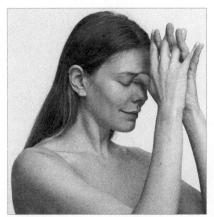

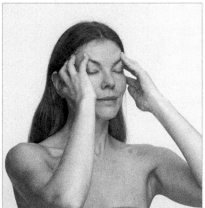

5. Brow lean: Interlace your fingers and place your thumbs under your brow bone. Lean your head forwards and hold for 10 seconds. Repeat three times.

6. Temple comb: Place four fingers onto your temples and slide your fingers towards your hairline. Repeat five times.

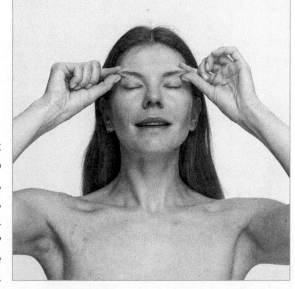

7. Brow pinch: Using your thumb and index fingers, pinch your brows, creating a little fold. Work your way along your whole brow twice.

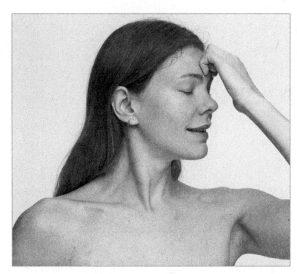

8. Knuckles on forehead: Using your knuckles, massage your forehead in a circular motion for 30 seconds.

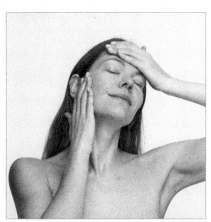

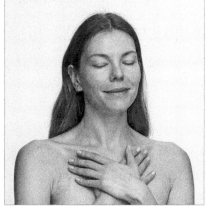

9. Sweeps: Using your palms, start sweeping from your forehead, down the sides of your face, finishing at your collarbones. Repeat three times on each side.

10. Deep release: Cross your wrists and place your palms over your chest. Take a deep breath in through your nose and exhale through your mouth with a 'Ha' sound, releasing any tension. Repeat three times.

Energizing Routine

If you're feeling a little low in energy and need a boost, this routine is for you. Regardless of the time of day or occasion, this five-minute pick-me-up can change the whole course of your day for the better. It incorporates invigorating, lifting movements to boost your energy and inspire. Experiment with speeding the movement up and have fun!

Products: cleanser, cream or oil

Time: 5 minutes

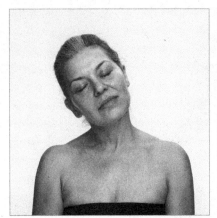 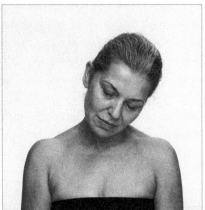

1. Neck roll: Keeping your shoulders wide, draw a large circle with your chin, rolling through your neck twice in each direction.

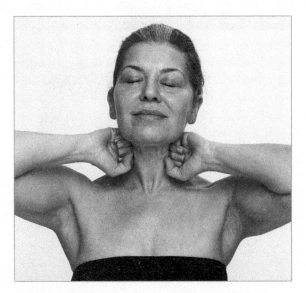

2. Knuckle circles: Place your fists onto each side of your neck and create a circular motion using the flat part of your knuckles, moving towards the back of your neck. Repeat five times.

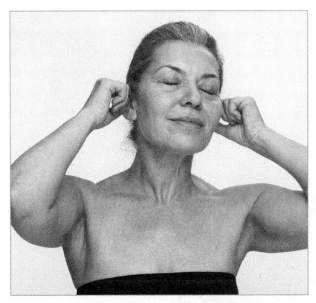

3. Ear massage: Using your fingers, massage both ears, releasing any tension.

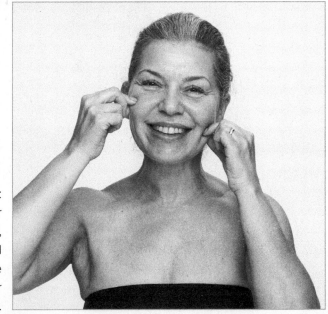

4. Pinching: Using your fingertips, lightly pinch all over your face and neck for 10 seconds.

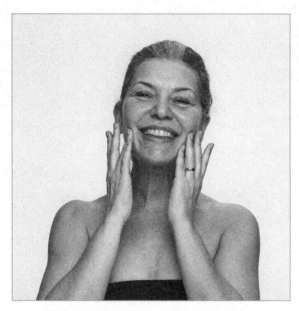

5. Tapping: Using your fingertips, gently tap across your whole face and neck for 10 seconds.

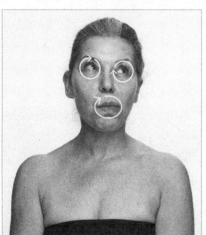
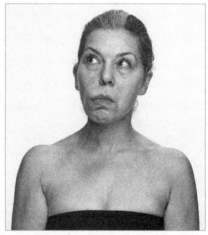

6. Eye and tongue circles: With your mouth closed, create circles with your tongue, pushing it out into the skin. At the same time, create circles with your eyes without moving your neck. Repeat five times in each direction.

7. Brow pinch: Using your thumbs and index fingers, pinch your brows, creating a little fold. Work your way along your whole brow twice.

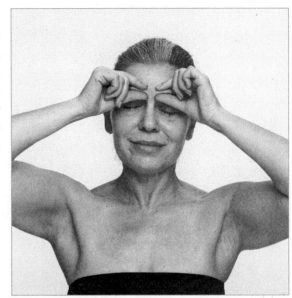

8. Forehead horizontal zigzag: Holding your index fingers horizontally on your forehead, create a zigzag motion by pushing your fingers towards each other and then away from each other, moving across your whole forehead.

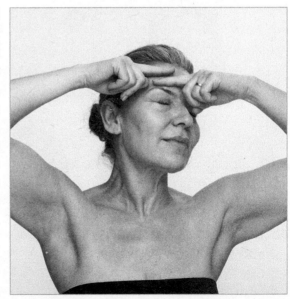

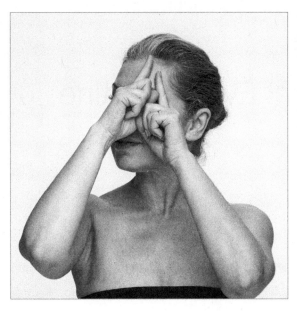

9. Forehead vertical zigzag: Create the same movement as above, but holding your fingers vertically this time.

K'S TIP

Massaging the ears and the area around them has countless benefits:

- It helps to release tension in the head, temples and forehead.

- It helps to improve the oval of the face and sculpt the jawline.

- It promotes relaxation and relieves stress.

- It improves circulation and helps to de-puff the face.

- It promotes lymphatic drainage and removes toxins.

- It improves the appearance of lines and wrinkles.

Special Event Routine

This massage is all about revealing your natural glow and radiance, helping you to achieve a lifted, sculpted look and to accentuate the natural contours of your face. If you're getting ready for an important event or simply want to look your best for a special occasion, do this the night before. If the event is today, there's still time. Think of this routine as a natural glow-up. By boosting blood flow and stimulating the tissues, we have the power to improve skin tone and achieve a more sculpted look.

Products: cleanser or cream

Time: 5–10 minutes

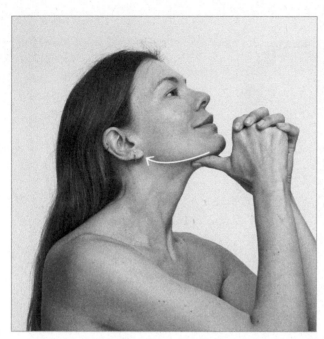

1. Sculpted jawline: Interlace your fingers and place your thumbs under your chin. Slide your thumbs along your jawline all the way towards your ears. Repeat five times.

2. Jawline hook: Curl all your fingers in, leaving your thumbs out. Place your thumbs under your chin, pressing your index fingers to your jawline. Slide out from your chin towards your ears. Repeat five times.

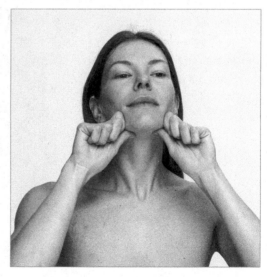

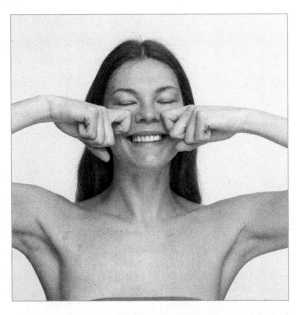

3. Cheek hook: Keeping your index fingers curled, place them on either side of your nose. Slide out towards your ears. Repeat five times.

4. Forehead hook: Place your curled index fingers in the middle of your forehead, then slide them out towards your temples. Repeat five times.

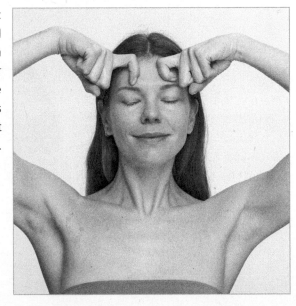

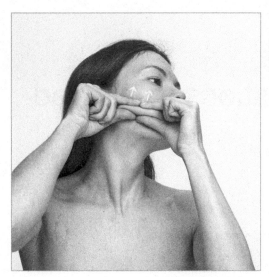

5. Skin rolling: Using your thumbs and index fingers, create a fold of skin at your jawline and start rolling it up your cheek. Repeat four times.

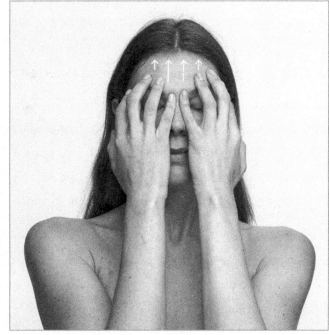

6. Brow lift: Place four fingers of each hand above your brows and slide up towards your hairline five times.

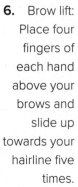

Your Questions Answered

Q. My skin looks flushed after a massage. Is that normal?

A. Yes, this is completely normal. Massage stimulates blood flow, which will create some redness on the skin. If you find that your skin gets overly red when massaging, try using less pressure or a different product.

Q. Why am I getting breakouts since I started massage?

A. There could be several reasons for this. First, you might be using the wrong product. If you have congestion-prone skin, massaging while cleansing might be a better option for you (*see page 35*). Alternatively, refer back to page 38 to find the right oil for you. Also, make sure to wash your face and hands prior to massage, as well as after.

Second, your body could be detoxing. Massage stimulates skin cell turnover, so your skin starts to purge. If you're already being mindful of cleanliness and using the right products, give it time and make sure to drink plenty of water to aid this detoxification process.

Q. How long will the results of facial massage last?

A. The results of a facial massage can last from 72 hours up to a week or even longer, depending on the individual and how consistent you are with it. To maintain optimal skin health and see long-term results, I recommend practising regularly.

Q. I feel very tired and sluggish after the lymphatic drainage massage. Is that normal?

A. Completely. Some people feel energized and elated after a massage and some feel sleepy and drained. This all depends on how well your lymphatic system is functioning. If you've never practised manual lymphatic drainage and self-massage, your system might be slightly stagnant and in need of some extra love and attention. Keep going and drink plenty of water after a self-massage to help flush out toxins and aid detoxification.

Q. Can I combine several routines together?

A. The routines in Part II are all designed to be a complete massage in themselves. You can, however, practise one in the morning and a different one in the evening, adding the warm-up routine on page 61 before each of those. The routines in Part IV, which address target areas, can be mixed and matched.

PART III

FACE MASSAGE FOR COMMON FEELINGS AND CONCERNS

In this part, we'll address some common feelings, concerns and insecurities you might be experiencing and perhaps feel overwhelmed by. I hope the following routines will become your go-to tools to move through those feelings and come out the other side feeling lighter, more confident and ready for whatever is next.

You can perform these routines anytime you feel like it. Work your way through them one by one and try to notice which ones feel particularly good to you. Maybe they will become your favourite massages to include in your morning, evening or even midday routine.

Don't forget to start with the warm-up sequence on page 61 before doing any of the following routines.

Feeling Puffy

We've all been there – a little too much salt (or wine), a little cry at a sad movie or feeling congested and under the weather and it seems that your eyes and face feel quite puffy, your belly feels a little bloated and your legs feel heavy. This routine will stimulate lymphatic drainage, which will help clear any blockages and accelerate the flow of fluids, as well as release any fluid build-up around the eyes and cheeks. Even though we're working primarily on the face here, stimulating your lymph flow will have a profound and positive effect on your whole lymphatic system.

I recommend doing this massage standing, as being upright will encourage fluid to drain from the face and any swelling to reduce quickly.

Products: cleanser, cream or oil applied all over the face and neck

Time: 8–10 minutes

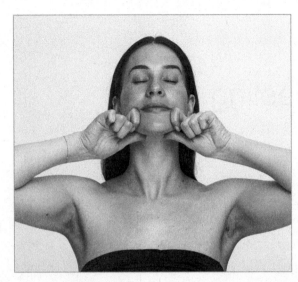

1. Jawline hook: Curl all your fingers in, leaving your thumbs out. Place your thumbs under your chin, pressing your index fingers to your jawline. Slide out from your chin towards your ears. Repeat five times.

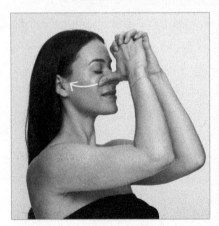

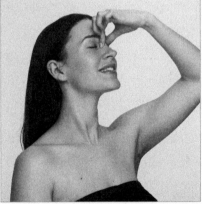

2. Cheekbone sculpt: Interlace your fingers and place your thumbs on either side of your nose. Slide your thumbs under your cheekbones towards your ears. Repeat five times.

3. Nose bridge pinch: Using your index finger and thumb, massage the bridge of your nose, moving up and down. Repeat five times.

4. Mouth release: Using your index fingers, massage the space on the outside of your nostrils in a circular motion. Repeat five times.

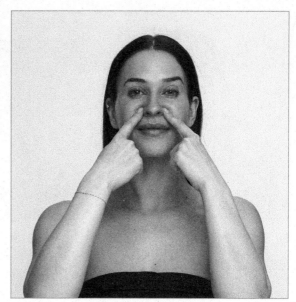

5. Pressure points: Place three fingers onto the bony part under your eyes. Close your eyes and gently press five times.

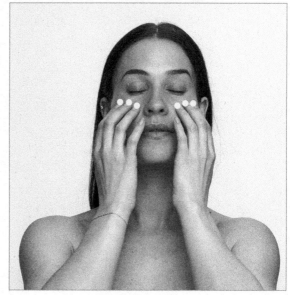

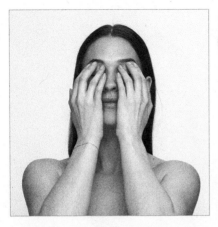

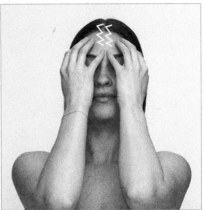

6. Pressure points: Place three fingers under your brow onto the edge of your brow bone. Close your eyes and gently press five times.

7. Scalp zigzag: Using your fingertips, move from your forehead into your hair in a zigzag motion, going side to side. Repeat across the whole head for about two minutes.

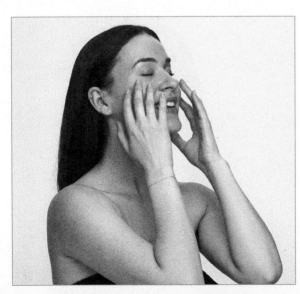

8. Tapping: Using your fingertips, gently tap across your chest and the sides of your neck and face for 10 seconds.

Feeling Tired

You've had a long day, a long week or have no energy to get on with the day – don't worry, I hear you! There are times when all I want to do is stay wrapped up in a blanket on the sofa with my dog, oblivious to the jobs and tasks that await me. And sometimes that's exactly what you should do, but if you want to shift that mood and boost your energy levels, let's begin. This routine increases the blood flow in the body, but also the flow of *Qi*, our vital force, which can help us feel more energized.

Products: clean skin, no product

Time: 5–8 minutes

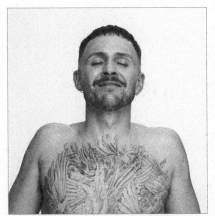 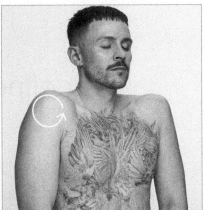

1. Shoulder rolls: Circle your shoulders five times forwards and five times backwards.

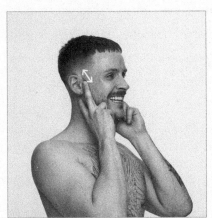 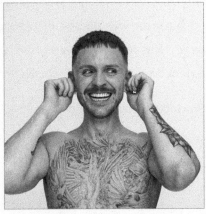

2. Peace fingers: Place your index fingers behind your ears and your middle fingers in front of your ears. Gently press up and down and create a rubbing movement. Repeat five times.

3. Ear massage: Using your fingers, massage your ears all over for 10 seconds.

4. Eye and tongue circles: With your mouth closed, create circles with your tongue, pushing it out into the skin. At the same time, create circles with your eyes without moving your neck. Repeat five times in each direction.

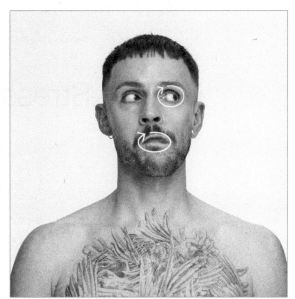

5. Pinching: Using your fingertips, lightly pinch all over your face and neck for 10 seconds.

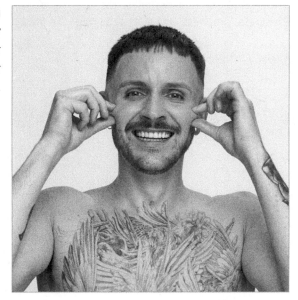

Feeling Stressed

As we explored in Part I, stress has a big impact on the body and can be overwhelming and all-consuming (*see page 22*). Whatever's causing that feeling, take a deep breath and massage any tension and worries away. With every touch and glide of your hand, feel the stress melt away. Shed everything you don't need. Move slowly and take your time.

Products: cream or oil applied all over the face and neck

Time: 10–15 minutes

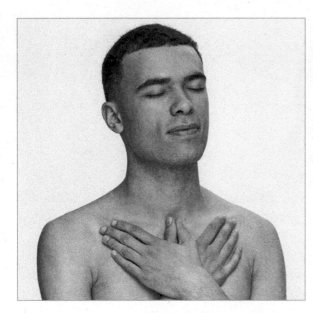

1. Deep release: Cross your wrists and place your palms over your chest. Take a deep breath in through the nose and exhale through the mouth with a 'Ha' sound, letting go of any tension. Repeat three times.

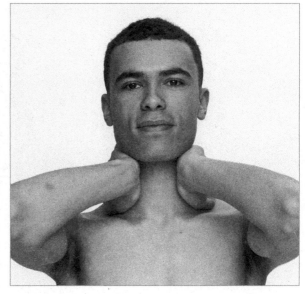

2. Speak your truth: Place the heels of both palms on either side of your neck close to the front, with your fingers facing back. Slide your palms back four times.

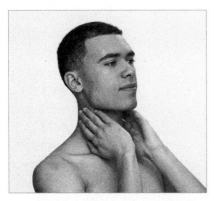
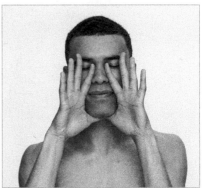

3. Lymphatic drainage: Place your palms under your ears on either side of your neck. Gently slide your palms down towards your collarbones. Repeat four times.

4. Butterfly: With your thumbs under your chin, frame your mouth and nose with your index fingers, opening out your palms. Slide your hands out to the sides of your face, gently pressing your index fingers onto your face. Repeat five times.

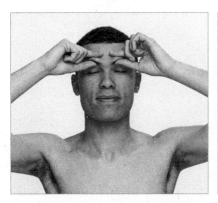
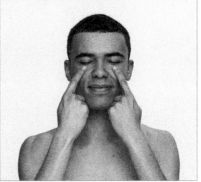

5. Brow pinch: Using your thumb and index fingers, pinch your brows, creating a little fold. Work your way along your whole brow twice.

6. ST2 pressure point: Place the tips of your index fingers directly below your pupils, approximately two fingers width down. Gently press and release five times.

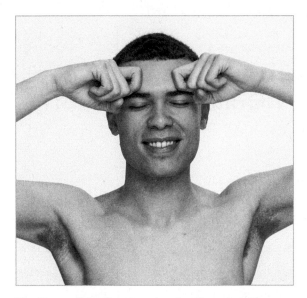

7. Brow slide: Create a hook with your index fingers. Meet your knuckles in the centre of your forehead and slide them out towards your temples. Repeat five times.

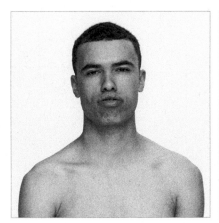 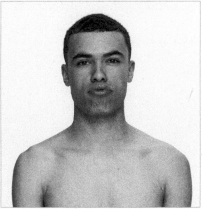

8. Lip flutter: Take a breath in and, as you exhale, flutter your lips.

Feeling Headachy

Headaches can occur for countless reasons. If you prefer a natural remedy to a painkiller, the simple steps in this routine will find your trigger points and relieve any pain around your head, temples, neck and shoulders. Try to create a calm, quiet atmosphere with soft or dimmed lighting. Maybe light a candle or your favourite incense. Treat this time as a self-healing practice. Visualize the headache as water or a cloud leaving your body as you perform this massage.

Products: clean skin, no product

Time: 8–10 minutes

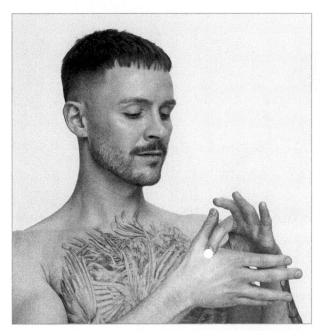

1. Pressure point LI-4: Firmly press into the space between the base of your thumb and index finger for five seconds. Repeat on the other side.

2. Back of the neck: Using both hands, massage the back of your neck in circular motions for 30 seconds.

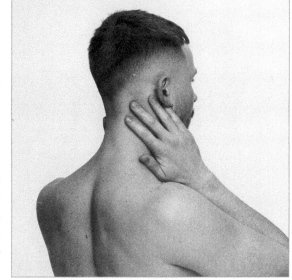

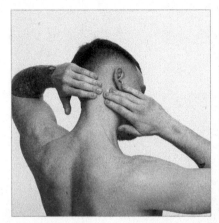

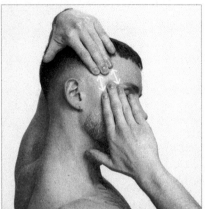

3. Base of the skull massage: Using your fingertips, massage the space below your skull at the back of your neck for 30 seconds.

4. Temples release: Placing one hand above the other with your fingertips facing in, gently pull your temples apart by moving your hands in opposite directions. Repeat five times on each side.

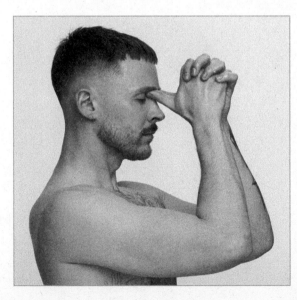

5. Brow lean: Interlace your fingers and place your thumbs under your brow bone. Lean your head forwards and hold for 10 seconds. Repeat three times.

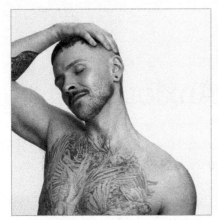 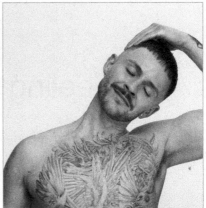

6. Neck stretch: Place one hand on top of your head and lean your head towards your elbow. Hold the stretch for five seconds. Repeat on the other side.

K'S TIP

Massaging the inner corners of your eyes can help to reduce tension and congestion. It's the location of a large muscle connection, where tension and pressure can build.

Feeling Anxious

It may be that you have an important meeting looming, a conversation to be had that makes your stomach turn or maybe an overwhelming anxiety about a growing to-do list. Let's get comfortable and move through that anxiety to come out feeling brighter and lighter. While doing this routine, try to focus your thoughts inwards on your strengths and the qualities you love about yourself. Allow that inner strength to help guide you through whatever is creating the anxiety.

Products: clean skin, no product

Time: 10 minutes

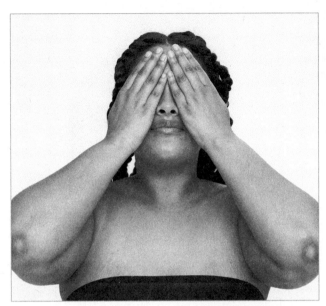

1. Breathe: Place your palms on your eyes and take three deep breaths. Try to lengthen the exhalation each time you breathe out.

2. Platysma stretch (*see the image on page 49 for reference*): Place your palms crossed on your chest. Stretch your chin up to the sky and hold for five seconds. Repeat three times.

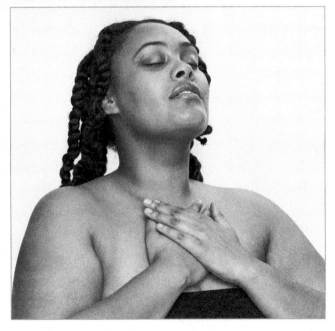

3. Side platysma stretch: Place one hand on the opposite side of your chest, just below your shoulder, palm down. Turn your head away from your hand. Stick your tongue out and up and move it from side to side, as if you are trying to lick your top lip. Continue for 10 seconds. Repeat on the other side.

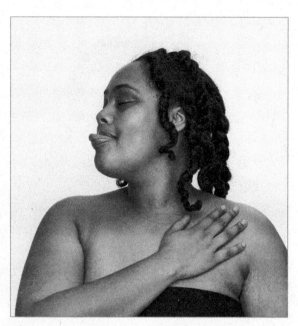

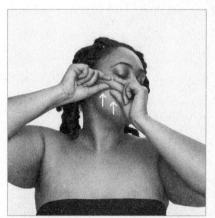

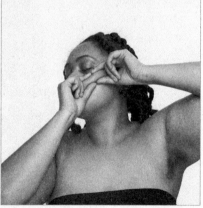

4. Sculpt and lift: Place your index fingers on top of your cheekbones. Hold them still. Use your thumbs to pull the skin from your jawline up towards your index fingers. Repeat five times on each side.

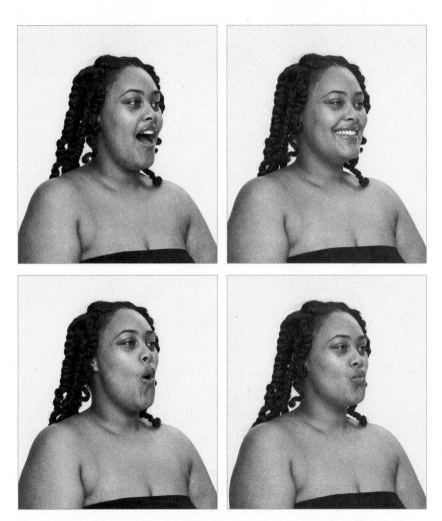

5. A-E-O-U: Open your mouth and say 'A, E, O, U.' Repeat all four letters five times.

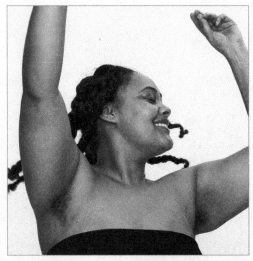

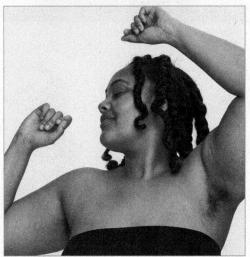

6. Shake it off: Do this standing. Close your eyes and just dance and shake off any tension that you might be holding on to.

Feeling Down

Sadness, heartache, loneliness, disappointment... whatever it is that's coming up for you, the only way to heal it is to feel it. So, allow yourself compassion and time, and give some love back to yourself. This routine allows you to release tension in the areas that tend to store negative emotions and physical pain. Use visualization while practising the routine; focus on memories that bring you the feeling of peace and joy.

Products: oil, applied over the neck and face

Time: 10 minutes

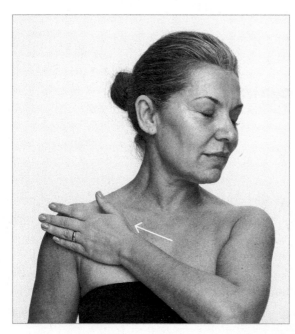

1. Chest massage: Place the heel of your palm next to your breastbone (at the centre of your chest) and slide your palm out towards your opposite shoulder. Repeat three times on each side.

2. Top of the arms: Cross your arms and massage the tops of your arms and shoulders with your palms. Imagine giving yourself a loving hug while you're doing it.

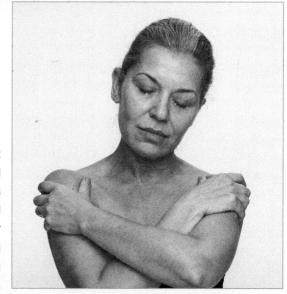

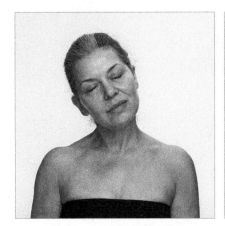 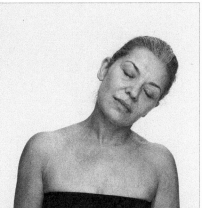

3. Neck circles: Gently circle your neck in both directions five times.

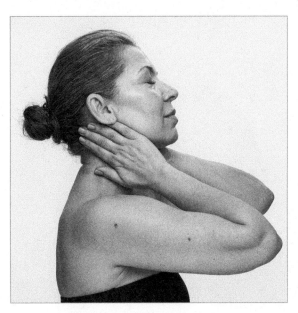

4. Behind the ears massage: Using your palms and fingers, massage the space behind your ears in a circular motion for 10 seconds.

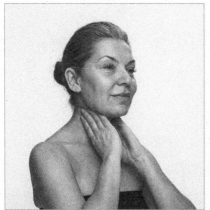 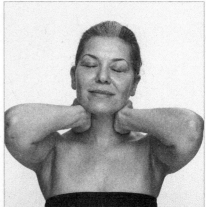

5. Neck sweep: Meet the heels of your palms with your fingers on the sides of your throat, facing towards the back. Slide your palms towards the back of your neck. Repeat five times.

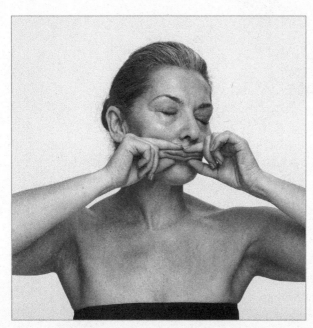

6. Lip massage: Using your thumbs and index fingers, massage your lips, pinching both lips together. Repeat along the whole mouth.

Your Questions Answered

Q. Sometimes massage makes me feel emotional and sad. Is that normal?

A. Completely! I feel you and I'm sending you love. Feelings and emotions often come up when we turn our attention inwards – the heightened awareness can bring things to the surface. Your physical body stores trauma, and massage can shift those blockages and stagnation and give you an opportunity to release. Remember, the only way is through. So feel what you need to feel and allow the emotions to wash over you.

Q. Can I massage if I'm not feeling well?

A. Unlike contact massage from a therapist, self-massage has no limits. So, especially when you're feeling under the weather, self-massage can be a fantastic natural remedy to assist with recovery. It helps flush out the toxins and promotes lymphatic drainage, which is linked to your immune system (*see pages 15–17*). It also restores the spark that you may have lost while you were covered in blankets and surrounded by boxes of tissues.

PART IV

FACE MASSAGE FOR TARGET AREAS

In this fourth and final part, we'll explore some routines that target a specific area of concern or one you'd simply like to focus on. This section was very much inspired by all the video requests I receive on my social media. I've focused on the areas that come up the most – from frown lines and nasolabial folds to forehead lines, jowls and more. You can perform these massages three to four times a week as a stand-alone routine or add them to any of the previous routines in Parts II and III.

I've also included face and eye yoga in this section (*see pages 191–7*). Face yoga, unlike massage, doesn't require much movement from your hands and targets muscles to tone, rather than lengthen and soften, so it works amazingly well in combination with the massage routines. Think of face and eye yoga as a visit to the gym, and the massage routines as like stretching and yin yoga.

As always, remember to do the warm-up sequence on page 61 before you get started.

Chest and Neck Lines

The chest and neck areas are often neglected when it comes to skincare application and massage. However, they're also the first areas that reveal our lifestyle and any signs of ageing. It's therefore important to give them some love and take your skincare all the way down to your breasts. By doing so, you can improve skin elasticity, minimize lines, achieve better tone and also have a positive effect on your posture.

CHEST LINES

Working with deeper tissues and muscles in the chest helps with better posture, more open breathing and your shoulder position. As busy, driven people we spend a lot of time leaning over laptops, books and phones with our shoulders rounded forwards. This means the muscles in our upper back are lengthening, while the muscles in our chest area are shortening. This, in turn, creates lines and loosening of the skin. Massaging the chest helps to open it up, reduce those wrinkles and improve the elasticity of the skin. Breathe deeply and enjoy this routine.

Products: oil, cream or even body lotion

Time: 5 minutes

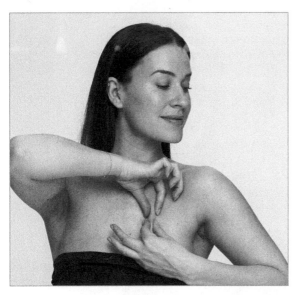

1. Double pinch and roll: Using both hands, create a fold of skin with your thumbs and index fingers next to your breastbone and roll that fold all the way towards your armpit. Repeat three times on each side.

2. Single pinch and roll: Using one hand, create a fold of skin with your thumb and index finger next to your breastbone and roll that fold all the way towards your armpit. Repeat three times on each side.

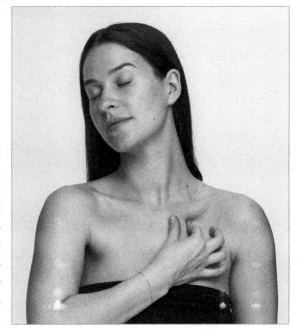

3. Chest massage: Place the heel of your palm next to your breastbone and slide your palm out towards your opposite shoulder. Repeat three times on each side.

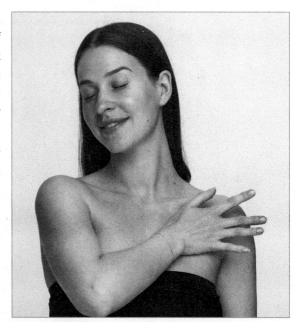

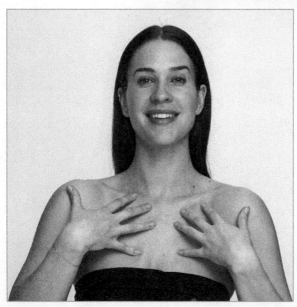

4. Chest circles: Using your fingers, create circular motions around the chest, working from the centre outwards. Repeat five times.

NECK LINES

If you spend a lot of time at a desk, the chances are you're relaxing into a rounded back with a chin dropped to your chest. This has a negative effect on your overall posture and builds tension in the neck and even in the back of the skull causing pain, headaches and tension. Massaging the neck not only improves lines and wrinkles, but also has a wonderful effect on your posture and reduces tension and aches in the upper body.

Products: oil or cream

Time: 5 minutes

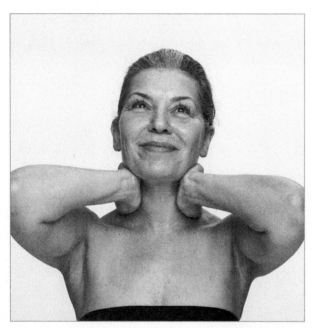

1. Neck sweep: Meet the heels of your palms with your fingers on the sides of your throat, facing towards the back. Slide your palms back towards the back of your neck. Repeat five times.

2. Knuckles on neck: Create fists with your hands and, using your knuckles, massage the sides of your neck in a circular motion for 30 seconds.

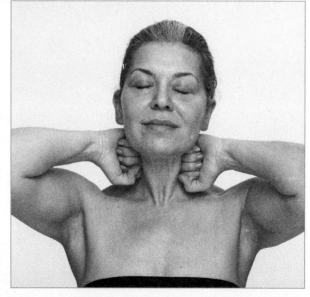

3. Venus pinch: Venus rings are the horizontal lines that appear on the neck, in the form of circles. Locate a horizontal line on your neck. Gently pinch the area of the line and rub it between your fingers. Move along the whole line, working in both directions. Repeat on all lines that are visible.

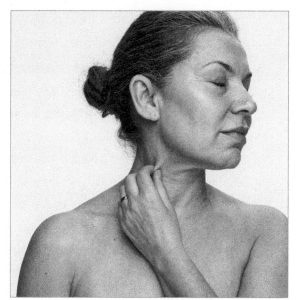

4. Side platysma stretch: Turn your head to one side. Stick your tongue out and up and move it from side to side, as if you are trying to lick your top lip. Continue for 10 seconds. Repeat on the other side.

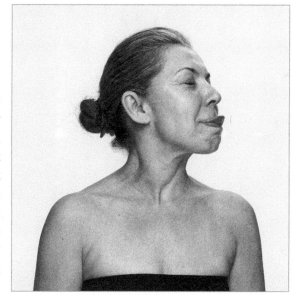

THE PLATYSMA

This is one of my favourite muscles in the body. Working with it has a profound effect on not just your face, but also your neck, shoulders, chest and even back. By lengthening and releasing the platysma muscle, we can minimize lines and wrinkles, reduce a double chin and jowls and define the oval of the face. Stagnation and tension in this muscle can also affect your lymphatic health – when the lymph is not draining efficiently it can lead to puffiness, water retention, dullness and dark circles around the eyes. The platysma muscle contributes to facial expressions, swallowing and speech (*see page 47*). Strengthening it can prevent sagging skin and enhance facial tone, while supporting natural movements and reducing the risk of neck stiffness or discomfort.

The Lower Face

The following massages focus on the lower third of the face. With a combination of these routines, you can achieve a more sculpted look in the oval of the face and also reduce tension in your jaw, neck and shoulders. If you grind or clench your teeth, these are also for you.

DOUBLE CHIN

Did you know that in Chinese medicine, your chin corresponds to your hormonal and reproductive system, and massaging this area has a positive effect on both? Besides the invisible benefits, chin massages can also help reduce double chins and wrinkles, and encourage smoother skin and better elasticity. This routine is a combination of massage and face yoga to sculpt and lift, but also strengthen the surrounding muscles to tone the area. When practising this exercise, think about the position of your tongue when you swallow.

Products: oil or cream

Time: 5–8 minutes

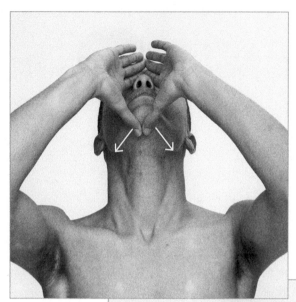

1. Thumb sculpt: Place the pads of your thumbs under your chin and slide them towards your ears following your jawline. Repeat five times.

2. Thumbs stretch: Place the pads of your thumbs under your jawline on one side and slide them away from each other. Repeat five times on each side.

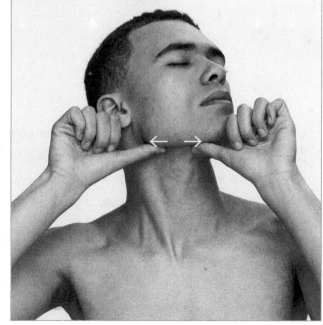

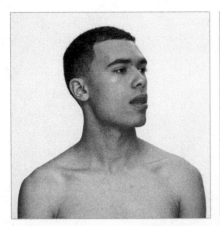
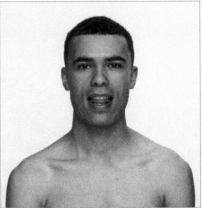

3. Tongue press: Keeping your mouth and jaw relaxed, try to press the root of your tongue to the roof of your mouth. Imagine swallowing. Repeat 20 times.

4. Tongue clicks: Create a clicking sound with your mouth by sliding your tongue along the roof of your mouth. Repeat 20 times.

THE TONGUE

Your tongue is a muscular organ that's made up of group of muscles. Its primary job is, of course, to manipulate food and aid swallowing, but weakness in these muscles, as well as improper position of the tongue, can also contibute to the appearance of a double chin and sagging jawline. This is why we need to exercise our tongues!

JAWLINE SCULPT

This is a super-simple routine that's as relaxing as it is visually beneficial. Make sure to breathe deeply and keep your shoulders relaxed throughout. We work with skin and deeper tissues to create a lifting muscle memory, reduce water retention to de-puff and to tone the jaw and chin area.

Products: oil or cream

Time: 5–8 minutes

1. Jawline hook: Curl all your fingers in, leaving your thumbs out. Place your thumbs under your chin, pressing your index fingers to your jawline. Slide out from your chin towards your ears. Repeat five times

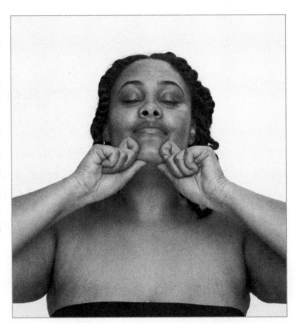

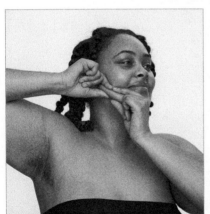 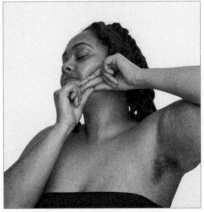

2. Skin rolling: Place your thumbs under your jawline. Create a fold between your thumbs and index fingers and start rolling and pinching the skin up towards your cheekbones. Move from your ear all the way towards your nose, working one section at a time.

146

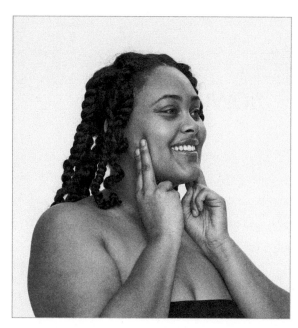

3. Beauty angle: Using your index and middle fingers, massage the corners of your jawline and chewing (masseter) muscle in circular and up-and-down movements (*see the image on page 49 for reference*). Repeat five times.

4. Chewing muscle release: Clench your hands into fists, open your mouth slightly and using your knuckles, massage the chewing (masseter) muscle pressing in and up and down. Continue for 30 seconds.

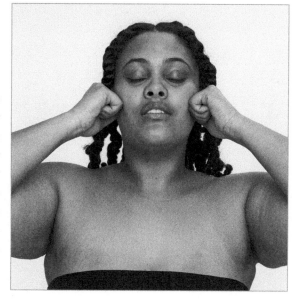

JOWLS

Jowls are pockets of loose skin and fat that can appear below the jawline. They're a completely natural sign of ageing, but can also be affected by weight fluctuation, smoking, bad posture and even dental work. This routine combines massage and face yoga to lift and tone the tissues and surrounding skin, as well as strengthen the weakened muscles.

Products: oil or cream

Time: 5 minutes

1. Smile lift: Using two fingers on either side of your mouth, slowly slide up from the jawline towards your nose, lifting the corners of your mouth. Repeat five times.

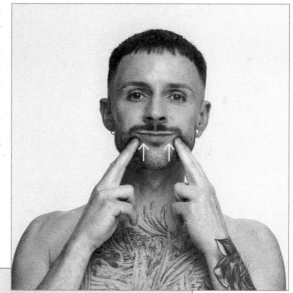

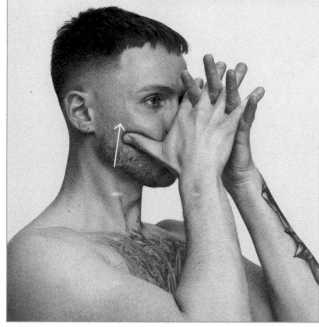

2. Side slide: Interlace your fingers, place your thumbs on your jawline and slide them up under your cheekbones. Repeat five times.

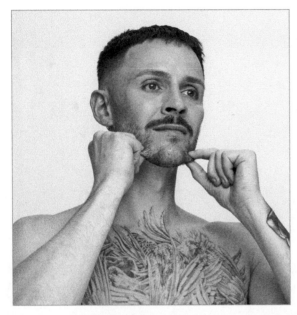

3. Jawline pinch: Using your thumbs and index fingers, pinch along your jawline. Continue for 10 seconds.

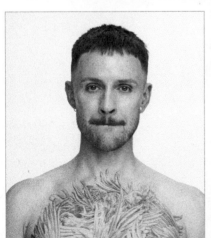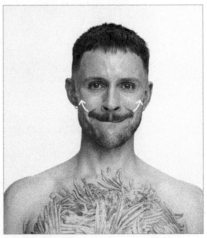

4. Lip curl: Curl your lips in around your teeth. Holding that position, try to lift the corners of your mouth up. Repeat 20 times, release and repeat 20 times again.

NASOLABIAL FOLDS

Nasolabial folds are deep lines that run diagonally from the outer edges of the nose to the sides of the mouth. Sometimes they can also blend in with marionette lines (which run from the corners of the mouth down to the chin), creating a sad, drooping facial expression. These lines can deepen with age, affected by lifestyle factors and poor posture. This massage works on lengthening and relaxing the muscles that we use repetitively to express emotions, which contribute to these folds.

Products: oil or cream

Time: 5–8 minutes

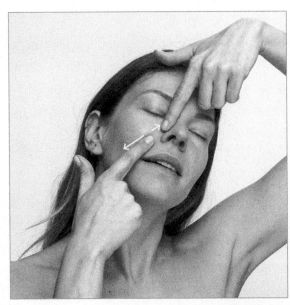

1. Muscle release: Place your index fingers diagonally into the nasolabial folds. Slide your fingers away from each other. Repeat five times on each side.

2. Turn and flick: Place the backs of your index fingers into the nasolabial folds. Turn your fingers out until your palms face towards your face and flick your fingers out. Repeat 10 times.

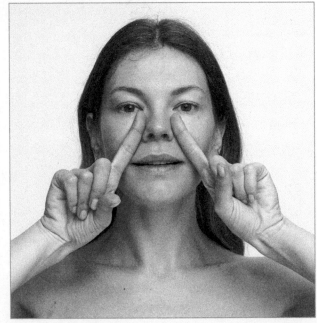

3. Pinch: Using your index fingers and thumbs, pinch the skin around the nasolabial folds. Repeat for 30 seconds.

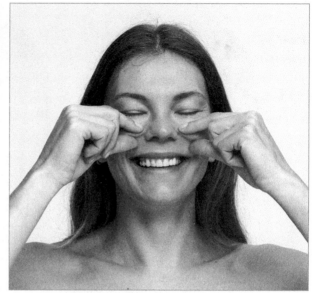

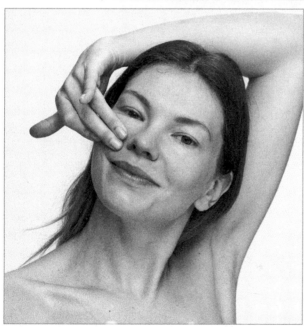

4. Spider fingers: Bring your arm over your head and, using two or three fingers, massage the fold by pulling it up and releasing it. Continue for 10 seconds on each side.

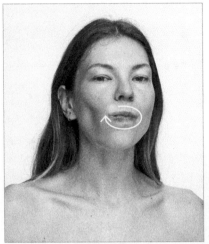 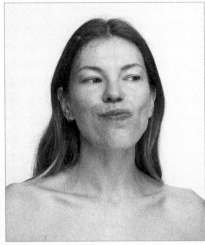

5. Tongue push: With your mouth closed, push your tongue out, moving in a circular motion. Continue for 10 seconds.

THE ZYGOMATICUS

This muscle directly contributes to nasolabial folds by pulling the skin and the cheeks in towards the nose, creating a crease (*see the image on page 49*). This routine is very effective in lengthening this muscle, as well as stimulating the area to promote collagen and elastin production.

MOUTH LINES

Mouth lines include the fine lines that can appear above the upper lip, as well as lines that form vertically from the corners of the mouth towards the jawline (also known as marionette lines). Habits like smoking or drinking through a straw can worsen these lines. This massage improves those fine lines, as well as releasing tension in the area.

Products: oil or cream

Time: 3–5 minutes

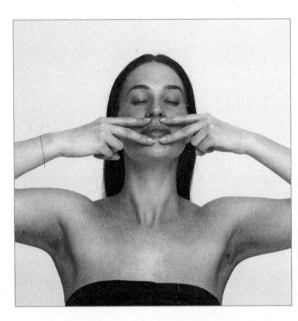

1. Peace sign sweep: Create the peace sign with your fingers. Place your index fingers above your lips and your middle fingers below. Slide them out from the centre of your lips 10 times.

2. Lip lines sweep: Using your index fingers, slide out from the middle of your lips. As you get to the nasolabial folds, flick your fingers out. Repeat 10 times.

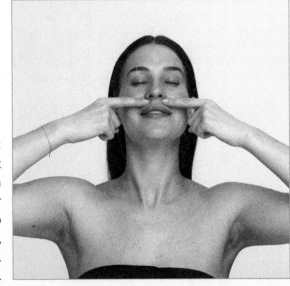

3. Depressor grab: Using your thumb and index finger, grab on to the depressor muscle (*see the image on page 49 for reference*). Make sure to grab on to the deeper layers and not just the skin, so try to create a fold of about ⅛ inch (4mm). Massage it by rubbing your fingers against each other. Repeat for 10 seconds on each side.

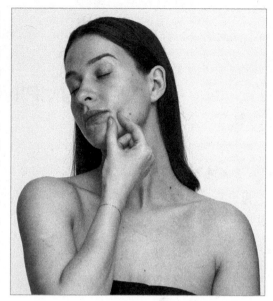

THE DEPRESSOR ANGULI ORIS

These muscles work by pulling the corners of the mouth down, so, when tensed, they shorten and permanently create a sad look on the face. We can lengthen them upwards and improve jowls, as well as lines in the mouth area.

LIP PLUMPING

This routine not only visibly plumps your lips, but also increases the flow of blood and nutrients to the surrounding tissues, promoting healthier skin and improved fine lines. It also helps to release the circular muscle of the mouth, an area where we can store tension and emotions, especially if you purse your lips when feeling anxious or stressed.

Products: clean skin, no product

Time: 3 minutes

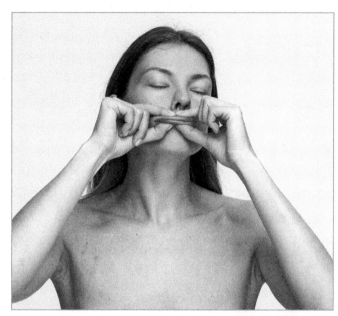

1. Lip massage: Using your thumbs and index fingers, massage your lips by pinching both lips together. Continue for 10 seconds.

2. Pinching: Using your index fingers and thumbs, pinch the lips and the space above and below. Continue for 20 seconds.

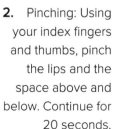
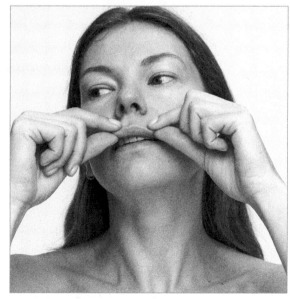

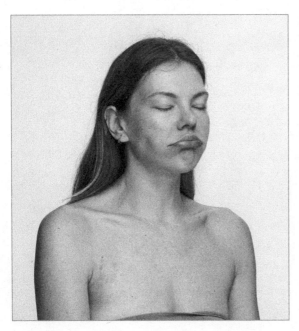

3. Fluttering: Take a breath in through your mouth and, as you exhale, flutter your lips. Repeat five times.

THE ORBICULARIS ORIS

This is a circular muscle of the mouth and is responsible for many mouth lines. Massaging it helps to improve lines, as well as plump our lips naturally.

The Middle Face

In this section, we'll focus on the chewing (masseter) muscle, as well as sculpting your cheekbones. We hold a lot of tension and emotion here – just think about all the movement that happens in this area alone... chewing and talking all day. But this is also our 'emotional area' – we can all relate to that feeling of clenched teeth when we're feeling anxious or angry. When not worked through, that emotion gets stored as tension in the muscles and can cause headaches, jaw pain, teeth grinding and neck and shoulder pain.

JAW TENSION AND CLENCHING

Teeth grinding, clenching, neck and shoulder pain, tension headaches and migraines can all be a result of tension in your jaw and the chewing (masseter) muscle. I myself used to suffer from TMJ (*see page 47*) and now my jaw pain is gone, I don't grind my teeth at night and the whole area feels lighter and softer. You can practise this routine every day.

Products: oil or cream

Time: 5–8 minutes

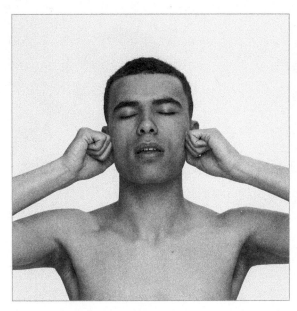

1. Knuckles massage: Clench your hands into fists. Open your mouth slightly and, using your knuckles, massage the chewing (masseter) muscle, pressing in and up and down (*see the image on page 49 for reference*). Continue for 30 seconds.

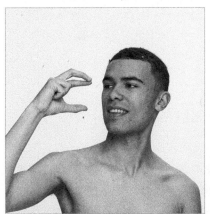 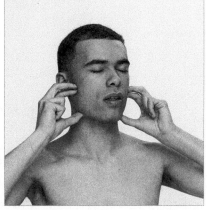

2. Jaw release: Place your middle finger on top of your index finger and, using your thumb, too, create a 'C' shape. Placing your thumbs under your jawline, press your index and middle fingers into your chewing muscle, making a circular movement. Work your way along the whole muscle, feeling for areas of tension.

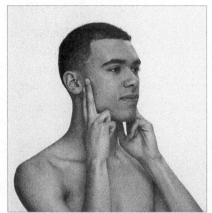

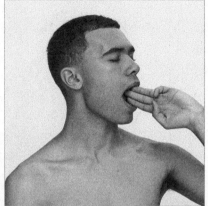

3. Joint massage: Using two fingers, massage the space in front of your ears, under your cheekbones, for 10 seconds.

4. Jaw stretch: Open your mouth and place a few fingers on top of one another, between your teeth. Hold for 10 seconds. Every time you practise this massage, try to progress to using more fingers, with the aim of lengthening the chewing muscle.

THE MASSETER

This is our hard-working chewing muscle, which is also an emotional muscle and is where we can store feelings and trauma. By releasing, softening and lengthening it we can reduce jaw clenching, neck pain and even headaches.

CHEEKBONE SCULPT

This massage is not just about achieving a lifted and sculpted look, it is also a fantastic release for an area where we tend to store a lot of tension. Try feeling right under the cheekbones and see if there are any knots or areas that feel tender or sore – gently massage into those areas with fingertips or knuckles.

Products: oil or cream

Time: 5–8 minutes

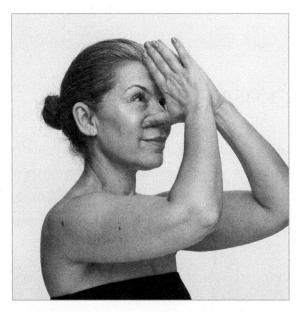

1. Cheekbone sculpt: Press your hands together and place your thumbs to each side of your nose. Slide your thumbs under your cheekbones towards your ears. Repeat five times.

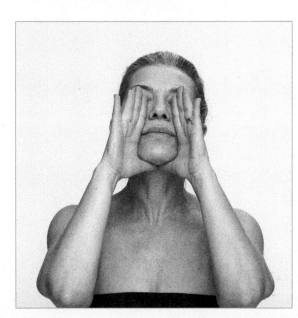

2. Butterfly: With your thumbs under your chin, frame your mouth and nose with your index fingers, opening out your palms. Slide your hands out towards the sides of your face, gently pressing your index fingers onto your face. Repeat five times.

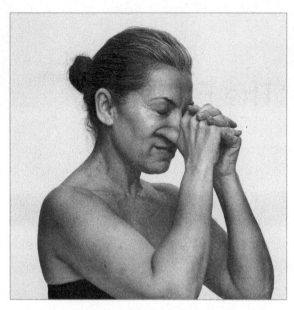

3. Tension release: Interlace your fingers and place your thumbs on each side of your nose, under your cheekbones. Slightly lean your head forwards. Hold for five seconds. Repeat three times.

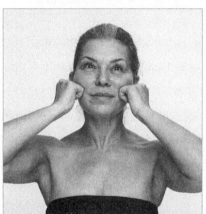

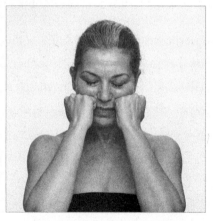

4. Knuckle scoop: Clench your hands into fists, then scoop your knuckles under your cheekbones from your nose all the way towards your ears. Repeat five times.

5. Knuckle lean: Create fists with your hands. Place your knuckles under your cheekbones and gently lean your head forwards. Hold for five seconds. Repeat three times.

The Eyes

They say that the eyes are the mirrors to our soul, but they're also often the mirrors to our internal and external wellbeing. Sayings like 'a twinkle in your eye' or 'dead behind the eyes' are descriptions and reflections of our emotional state. So working with your eye area can make a big difference to the overall brightness of your face.

It's important to remember that the skin around the eyes is thinner than the rest of your face, so a gentler, slower touch works best in this area. However, seeing the skin wrinkle a little as you perform the massages is totally okay. These massages also work really well when combined with the eye yoga routine on page 195, as you get to strengthen, lengthen and release, all at the same time.

PUFFY EYES

Puffiness around the eyes occurs as the structures supporting the eyelids weaken. The skin becomes thinner, the muscles relax and the normal fat that supports the eye can descend into the lower eyelid. Excess fluid can also pool in this area from water retention, poor lymph drainage and poor muscle function. This massage helps to promote the elimination of that fluid and encourage better lymph flow, which brightens and de-puffs the area.

We're going to use two spoons for this routine – my favourite handy tool! Pop them in the fridge or some cold water for at least 10 minutes before the massage for an extra cooling effect. Or dip them in hot water for five minutes before the massage for a soothing effect and if you're prone to dry eyes. Make sure to check the temperature of the spoons on the back of your hand before applying to your face.

Products: oil or cream, two spoons

Time: 8–10 minutes

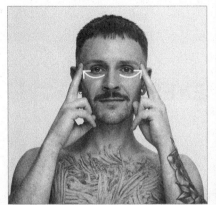 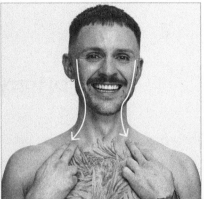

1. Lymphatic drainage: Using one or two fingers, sweep slowly and gently from the inner corners under your eye towards your ears, then down your neck, finishing above your collarbones. Repeat three times.

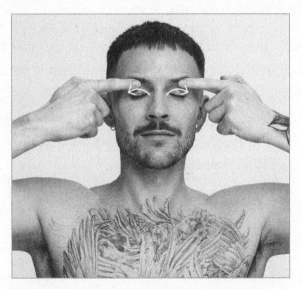

2. De-puffed lids: Using your index fingers, gently slide under your brows from the inner corner outwards. Repeat five times.

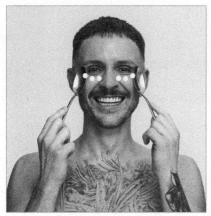 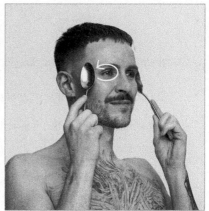

3. Spoon roll: Using the backs of the spoons, gently press them over the space under your eyes and roll them away from your nose. Repeat three times.

4. Spoon circles: Using the backs of the spoons, massage around your eyes in a circular motion. Repeat five times.

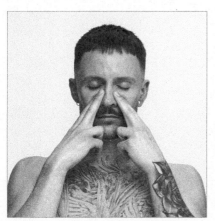 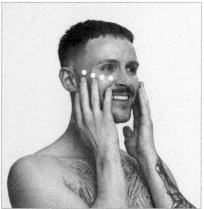

5. Congestion release: Using one or two fingers, massage the sides of your nose in a circular motion. Continue for 10 seconds.

6. Tapping: Using your fingertips, tap outwards under your eyes for 10 seconds.

K'S TIPS

Below are a few extra pointers for beautiful, healthy, bright eyes:

- Check your eyesight and wear appropriate glasses if required.

- Get enough sleep – this one is obvious, I know, but it's always worth a reminder.

- Make sure you wear sunscreen and apply it around the eyes, too.

- Apply a cold compress to your eyes regularly. You can use two cold spoons, cucumber slices or even used black tea bags left in the fridge for 10 minutes.

- A warm compress is also beneficial, especially if you suffer from dry eyes, as it stimulates the tear ducts that naturally lubricate the eyes. Warm spoons or tea bags are a wonderful choice.

DARK CIRCLES

One of the main reasons for dark circles is hyperpigmentation, which can be caused by both environmental factors (such as sun exposure, smoking and poor sleep) and genetics. However, fatigue, allergies, eye strain, dehydration and lifestyle factors can also contribute to darkness under the lower eyelids. As we age, we also experience a decrease in the fat and collagen that help to maintain the skin's elasticity. As this occurs, the dark blood vessels beneath our skin become more prominent, causing the area below our eyes to darken. Massage stimulates the blood flow and oxygenates the skin, resulting in a brighter and healthier appearance.

Products: eye or face cream

Time: 5–8 minutes

1. Eye circles: Using your middle (or index and middle) fingers, massage gentle circles around your eyes. Repeat five times.

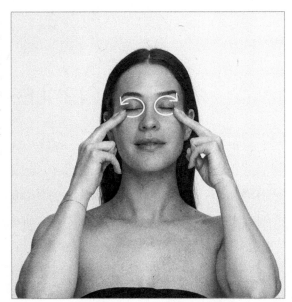

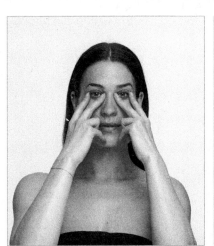
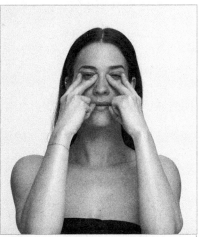

2. Squint: Place the pads of your index and middle fingers gently into the inner and outer corners of your eyes. Keeping your face relaxed and still, squint your eyes 20 times.

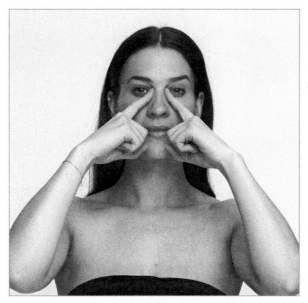

3. Inner corner massage: Using your index fingers, massage the inner corners of your eyes in a circular motion for 10 seconds.

4. Circle pinch: Using your thumbs and index fingers, gently pinch the skin around the eyes, moving in a circle. Continue for 10 seconds.

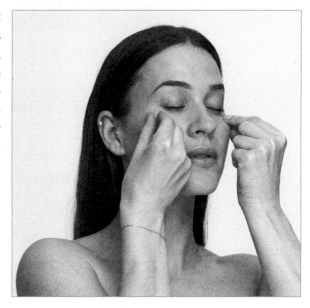

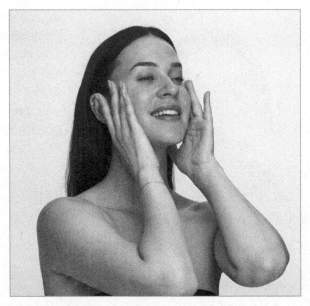

5. Tapping: Tap the pads of your fingers under and around your eyes for 10 seconds.

THE ORBICULARIS OCULI

This is a circular muscle that connects in the inner corner of the eye. Tension can pool in that area creating stagnation or fluid retention.

CROW'S FEET

Tension around the eyes and forehead, the natural process of ageing, dehydration and poor eyesight can all contribute to fine lines in the corners of our eyes. Use your favourite eye or face cream for this massage and use gentle strokes to de-puff, brighten and improve lines. The skin in this area is thin, so move slowly using gentle pressure.

Products: eye or face cream, one spoon

Time: 5 minutes

1. Peace sign pinch: Gently stretch the skin on your temples using peace sign fingers. With the other hand, pinch the area of crow's feet for 10 seconds.

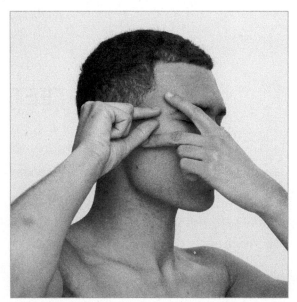

2. Temples release: Placing one hand above the other, with your fingertips facing in, gently pull apart your temples by moving your hands in opposite directions. Repeat five times on each side.

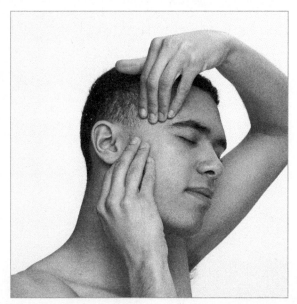

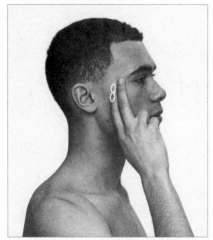 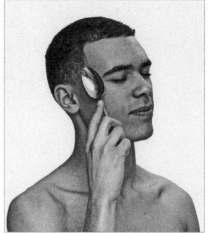

3. Figure of eight: Using one or two fingers, draw a figure of eight on your temples with your fingertips. Repeat five times.

4. Spoon circle: Using the back of the spoon, gently press down at your temple and move in small circles. Repeat for 10 seconds on each side.

THE TEMPORALIS

When the temporalis muscle is under tension, it shortens and creates creases in the outer corner of the eyes. Reducing tension in this muscle and lengthening it helps to reduce fine lines.

The Forehead

Whether they're horizontal or vertical, forehead lines are usually a sign of a particularly expressive forehead or a genetic predisposition. Worry, surprise, stress, anger or even poor eyesight all play a part in their appearance. Stimulating the tissues in this area and promoting blood flow acts like natural filler, as it helps to promote collagen and elastin production – the building blocks of our skin. Massage also helps to soften and relax those hard-working muscles that move all day to express our emotions.

FROWN LINES OR 'ANGRY 11S'

Overthinkers and deep thinkers unite! Ever caught yourself frowning without realizing? I've definitely been there. Tension in the area between the eyebrows, called the glabella, and contraction of the corrugator muscle (*see page 49*) not only creates lines in the area, but can also cause headaches and pains in the head. It's also the area that tends to reveal our stresses and emotions. The lines in this area are caused by repetitive facial expressions like smiling, frowning, laughing and even blinking.

This is a super-simple routine that works with deeper tissues and muscles to help combat the visibility of frown lines, lengthening and relaxing the muscles that pull our brows inwards and down. No product is required for this one – just use your fingers and some light pinches and pulls. This is my favourite massage after a day of overthinking and working hard. Breathe deeply and keep your shoulders down.

Products: clean skin, no product

Time: 8–10 minutes

1. Forehead hook: Place your curled index fingers in the middle of your forehead, then slide them out towards your temples. Repeat five times.

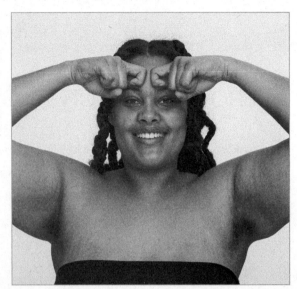

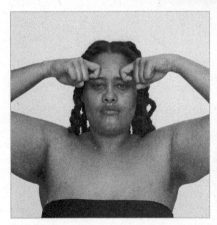

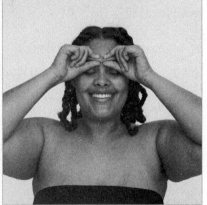

2. Hook and resist: Following the previous move, stop your fingers in the middle of your brow. Gently press down and try to frown, resisting the movement with your fingers. Repeat 10 times.

3. Brow fold: Using your thumbs and index fingers, create a fold of skin and muscle between the brows. Hold the tissues for five seconds. Keep your shoulders and face relaxed. Repeat five times.

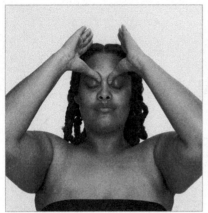

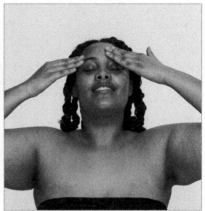

4. Brow lean: Place your thumbs under your brow bone. Lean your head forwards and hold for 10 seconds. You could even place your elbows on the table for extra support. Repeat three times.

5. Stroke and release: Using your fingers, gently stroke your forehead in an outwards motion. Continue for 10 seconds.

THE PROCERUS MUSCLE

This pulls our brows inwards and, when in tension, can create a permanent look of a crease or fold between the brows. We can open up this area and reduce lines by stretching and relaxing this muscle.

FOREHEAD LINES

This routine is a combination of massage and face exercises. By combining both and using your knuckles, you work with the deeper tissues and muscles of the face, softening forehead lines by releasing tension in the muscles and increasing blood flow.

Products: clean skin, no product

Time: 5 minutes

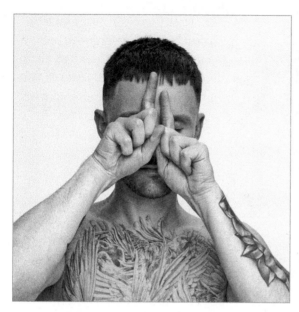

1. Vertical zigzag: Place your index fingers vertically in the middle of your forehead between your brows. Using the sides of your fingers, create a zigzag motion, moving them up and down. Move across the whole forehead, first in one direction, then the other, twice.

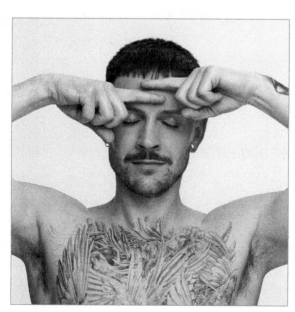

2. Horizontal zigzag: Place your index fingers horizontally across your forehead, your fingertips pointing inward. Using the sides of your fingers, create a zigzag motion, moving them from side to side. Move across the whole forehead, first in one direction, then the other, twice.

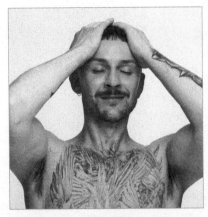

3. Hold and resist: Place your palms flat on your forehead over your brows. Firmly press down and hold the skin in place. Try to lift your brows, but resist the movement with your palms. Repeat 20 times.

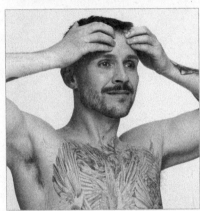

4. Forehead slide: Place the fingertips of both hands together in the centre of your forehead. Slide them away from each other, firmly pressing down as you slide. Repeat five times.

THE OCCIPITOFRONTALIS

Tension in the occipitofrontalis muscle - a sheet-like muscle on our forehead - not only creates lines but can also cause headaches and tension in the neck. This massage works with this muscle to release any tension.

The Scalp

One of my go-to massages after a long day or when I feel tension in my body is a scalp massage. There are many pressure points around the scalp that can help with relaxation and even reduce our blood pressure. Massaging the scalp has many benefits.

- It boosts blood circulation for radiant, glowing skin.

- It calms the nervous system and releases stress.

- It promotes natural hair growth by stimulating the hair follicle.

- It elevates sleep quality for restful nights.

- It reduces tension headaches.

- It promotes mindful relaxation by bringing us to the present moment.

- It nourishes scalp and hair health by strengthening the hair roots and nourishing hair shafts.

- It lifts and tones facial muscles.

- It encourages calmer breath and a more peaceful state.

HAIR-GROWTH MASSAGE

This massage is not just effective at stimulating hair growth, it's also incredibly relaxing. You can do this every day, any time of the day, to release tension in your head, neck and shoulders. Use a hair oil (castor or coconut are good choices) for extra benefit.

Products: hair oil or no product

Time: 8–10 minutes

1. Gentle pull: Grab a section of hair in each hand. Gently pull up and move in a circular motion creating movement in the skin of the scalp. Continue for 20–30 seconds.

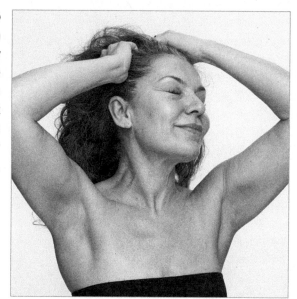

2. Scalp massage: Interlace your fingers. Using the heels of your palms, massage your head across the whole area of hair growth. Breathe deeply and keep your shoulders relaxed. Massage for one minute or longer.

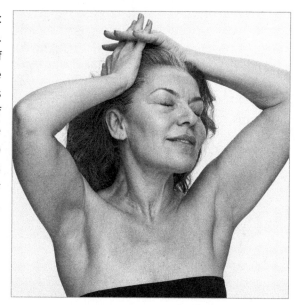

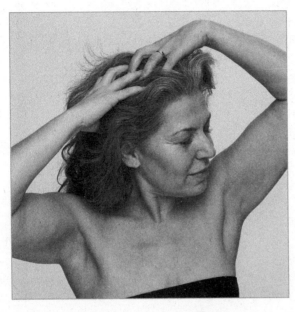

3. Zigzag: Using your fingertips, create a zigzag motion all across your scalp, especially focusing on areas that feel tender. Massage for 30–60 seconds.

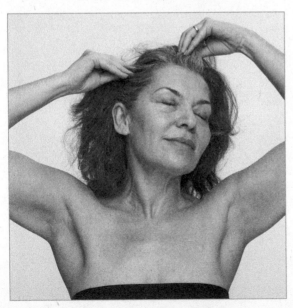

4. Pinching: Using your fingers, create a pinching motion all across the head. Continue for 60 seconds.

Face Yoga

Face yoga is different to face massage, as you use your facial muscles to perform the exercises, rather than keeping your facial muscles still and using your hands. It's a fantastic way to stretch and expand overused and tense muscles.

Our muscles lose their tone, as well as mass and volume, as we age. So you can also use face yoga as a gentle form of strength training for your face and neck to stimulate muscles to improve their tone and tightness.

Working out your muscles also increases circulation and blood flow, which creates a natural glow.

Products: clean skin, no product

Time: 5–8 minutes

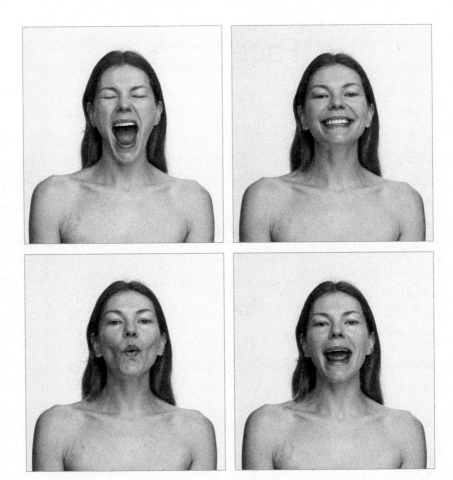

1. A-E-O-U: Open your mouth and say 'A, E, O, U.' Repeat all four letters five times.

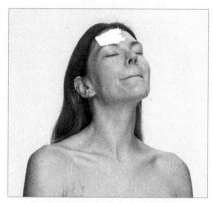 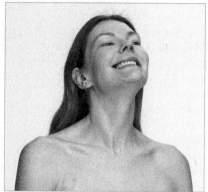

2. Platysma stretch 1: Curl your lips in around your teeth. Relax your shoulders and gently stretch your chin up to the sky. Hold for five seconds. Repeat three times.

3. Platysma stretch 2: Create a smile with your mouth, keeping your teeth together. Relax your shoulders and gently stretch your chin up to the sky. Hold for five seconds. Repeat three times.

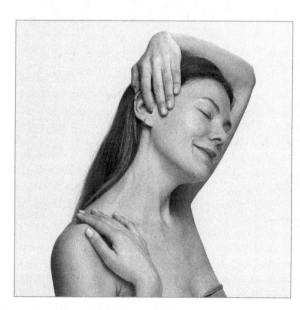

4. Side stretch: Drop your head to your left side. Place your left hand over your head, putting one finger inside the ear. Gently pull your left hand down and away from your right shoulder. Release and repeat five times before doing the same on the right side.

5. Tongue push: Keeping your mouth closed, push your tongue out, making a circular motion. Continue for 10 seconds.

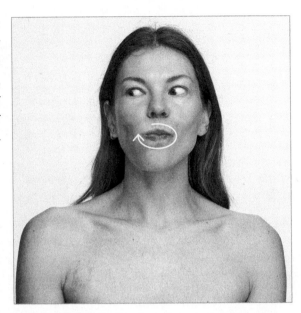

6. Hook and resist: Curl your index fingers to form a 'hook.' Place your index finger hooks in the middle of your brows. Gently press down and try to frown, resisting the movement with your fingers. Repeat 10 times.

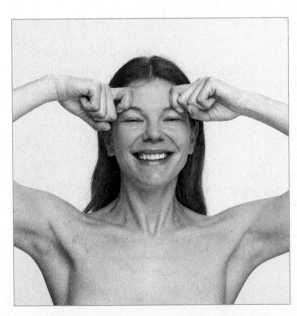

Eye Yoga

I do this routine every other day, sometimes in public places with my eyes closed. I have pretty bad vision and wear glasses or contact lenses, so I often feel tension in my eyes. This exercise gives my eyes a beautiful release, but it also has countless other benefits, like improving hooded eyelids and dark circles.

This routine can be done as a stand-alone or added to the face yoga routine (*see page 191*).

Product: clean skin, no product

Time: 5 minutes

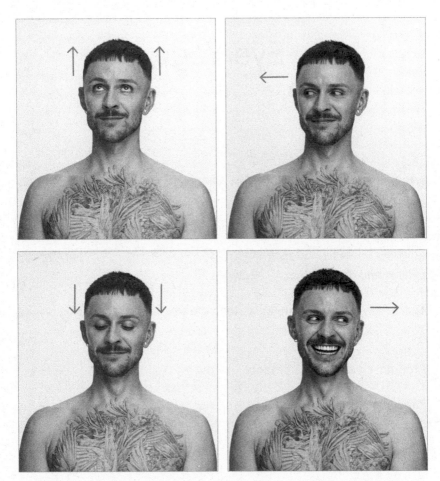

1. All directions: Keeping your head and face still, use the muscles of your eyes to look in all four directions, holding each for five seconds. Repeat four times.

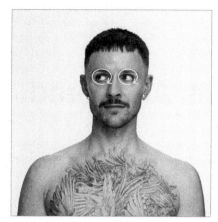

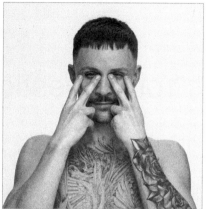

2. Circles: Keeping your head and face still, use the muscles of your eyes to circle them one way five times and then the other way five times.

3. Squint: Place the pads of your index and middle fingers gently into the inner and outer corners of your eyes. Keeping your face relaxed and still, squint your eyes 20 times.

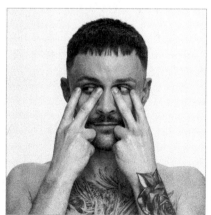

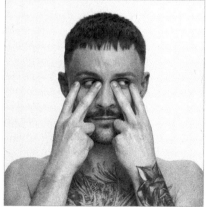

4. Squint side to side: Keeping your hands in the previous position, squint your eyes and look side to side 20 times.

Your Questions Answered

Q. Can I mix and match different target areas in one massage?

A. Yes, absolutely. These massages work very well combined together or added to the routines from Parts II and III.

Q. Can I do these a few times a day?

A. I wouldn't advise repeating massages on the same target area twice a day. More is not always better. Overstimulating the skin can cause congestion in some cases. Allow your skin and muscles the rest they deserve.

FINAL WORD

And here we are at the end of the book. First of all, I want to thank you for making it to these final pages and also for picking it up in the first place. Second, I want to congratulate you on making this investment in your health, wellness and personal peace.

Face massage has been a life-changing practice for me. It granted me the tools to better connect with my physical body, to understand it, listen to it intently and nourish it without needing a reason. I stopped waiting for symptoms and decided to provide my body with all the maintenance and care it needs. And I've never felt better. It also created a big shift in my emotional wellbeing. I feel more present and aware, less reactive and simply happier for introducing this meditative practice into my life.

I hope that this book will serve you as a tool and reminder that there are alternative holistic practices for beauty and wellness. Use it in the best way you see fit. Take what you need and if you're still left with questions or wanting more, don't hesitate to reach out. DM me on Instagram (@the_moments). I'll always do my best to get back to you and help.

Remember that self-care is soul care.

ENDNOTES

Part I: The Fundamentals

The Importance of Self-Care

P.5 The practice of massage has evolved over the years and new techniques are always being developed. For more on facial massage, see Sarfati, L. (2009), 'The Art and Science of Facial Massage': www.skininc.com/treatment/facial/article/21883421/the-art-and-science-of-facial-massage [Accessed 23 May 2024].

The Benefits of Face Massage

P.15. Understanding the lymphatic system and where the lymph nodes are allows for better purification of the skin. See Ozdowski, L. and Gupta, V. (2023), 'Physiology, Lymphatic System': www.ncbi.nlm.nih.gov/books/NBK557833/ [Accessed 24 September 2024].

P.15 The lymphatic system is an essential and often underappreciated component.... See MacGill, M. (2024), 'What Does the Lymphatic System Do?': www.medicalnewstoday.com/articles/303087 [Accessed 23 May 2024].

P.16 When your lymphatic system is functioning properly, you feel full of energy, clear-headed and ready to take on the world. See The Editors of Encyclopaedia Britannica (2024), 'Lymphatic System': www.britannica.com/science/lymphatic-system [Accessed 23 May 2024].

P.17 By stimulating the flow of lymph around the body with your two hands, you promote better circulation.... For more, see Stop Chasing Pain (2024), 'What is BIG 6TM?': www.stopchasingpain.com/the-big-6-tm/ [Accessed 23 May 2024].

P.17 ...one-third of all our lymph nodes are located from the neck up. See Banjar, F.K. and Wilson, A.M. (2022), 'Anatomy, Head and Neck, Supraclavicular Lymph Node.', www.ncbi.nlm.nih.gov/books/NBK544300/ [Accessed 24 September 2024].

P.20 ...face massage can actually improve the overall appearance of skin.... For more on lines and wrinkles, see Chesak, J. 'Decoding What These 7 Wrinkle Types Might Say About You' (2019), www.healthline.com/health/beauty-skin-care/wrinkles#wrinkle-types [Accessed 23 May 2024].

P.23 There are 11 organ systems in the body, and all of them suffer from prolonged exposure to stress. For more, see Stress Effects on the Body (2023), American Psychological Association: www.apa.org/topics/stress/body [Accessed 23 May 2024].

P.25 Research now shows that psychological stress negatively impacts the homeostasis, in other words, the balance and protective barrier of the skin. For more, see Garg, A., Chren, M.M., Sands, L.P., et al, 'Psychological stress perturbs epidermal permeability barrier homeostasis: Implications for the pathogenesis of stress-associated skin disorders', *Archives of Dermatology* (2001), 137(1): 53–9.

P.26 The brain–skin connection is a two-way street... For more, see Nathan, N. 2021), 'Stress May Be Getting to Your Skin, But It's Not a One-Way Street': www. health.harvard.edu/blog/stress-may-be-getting-to-your-skin-but-its-not-a-one-way-street-2021041422334 [Accessed 23 May 2024].

P.27 One of my go-to breathing techniques is the 4-7-8 breath. Developed by Dr Andrew Weil... For more on this, see www.drweil.com/videos-features/videos/breathing-exercises-4-7-8-breath [Accessed 3 October 2024].

P.28 When you touch something, the receptors on your skin send signals to your brain. For more on the somata-cognitive network, see Gordon, E.M., Chauvin, R. J., Van, A.N., et al (2023), 'A Somato-Cognitive Action Network Alternates with Effector Regions in Motor Cortex', *Nature*, 617: 351–9.

Getting Started

P.39 With an overwhelming, and even confusing, choice of facial oils, it can be hard to know how to pick the one that's right for you. See Herbal Dynamics Beauty (2023), 'Understanding the Comedogenic Scale for Oils and Butters': www. herbaldynamicsbeauty.com/blogs/herbal-dynamics-beauty/understanding-the-comedogenic-scale-for-oils-and-butters [Accessed 23 May 2024].

P.56 Did you know that contemplation is the second stage of the transtheoretical model (TTM)... For more, see Boston University School of Public Health (2022), 'The Transtheoretical Model (Stages of Change)': https://sphweb.bumc.bu.edu/otlt/mph-modules/sb/behavioralchangetheories/behavioralchangetheories6.html [Accessed 23 May 2024].

Part IV: Face Massage for Target Areas
Dark Circles

P.173 One of the main reasons for dark circles is hyperpigmentation... For more, see Anthony, K. (2024), 'What Causes Dark Circles Under Your Eyes?': www.healthline. com/health/dark-circle-under-eyes#age [Accessed 23 May 2024].

ACKNOWLEDGEMENTS

Many beautiful people made this book happen, so a quick thank you to:

Every client who's ever visited my studio and every person who's watched my videos and practised with me online. Thank you for the trust and motivation.

My mum and dad, for your unshakable belief and supporting hand through my life. Even when my ideas and plans sounded out of reach, you built those bridges in my mind of how to get there.

Nikita, my talented friend and photographer, whose beautiful work fills most pages of this book.

My beautiful friends Chris, Tegan and Rebecca, and to Monique and Dan, for appearing in this book and being the most wonderful models.

Susa, my illustrator extraordinaire and, above all, wonderful friend. I dreamed of having your work in my book and it's an honour to see it come to life.

Martina, my sweet, kind friend and guru of style and graphic design.

Oscar, my wonderful literary agent, for your trust, commitment, belief in me and support. This really wouldn't have happened without you.

Helen, my publisher, for your expert guidance, kindness and warmth.

Julia, my editor, your way with words is magic. Thank you for taking my mad professor scribbles and notes and translating them into these wonderful pages.

Leanne, Cathy and Lesley for your support and expertise in putting this book together.

Bryony and Jess, my agents and friends, you're the backbone to all my work and the support system I couldn't have done without.

And to my person, Matt. You're the fuel to my fire and the other half of my heart.

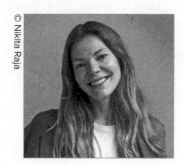

© Nikita Raja

About the Author

Ksenija Selivanova is a London-based facialist, facial massage expert and founder of the hugely popular **@TheMoments** YouTube channel. Having worked in the beauty and wellness industry, including with leading international, skincare and beauty brands, for many years, she has a fully rounded approach to feeling and looking well. A naturopathic nutritionist-in-training, Ksenija has also taught Pilates for many years. Working with clients in her beauty studio, as well as constant feedback and requests from her online students and audience, all inspired her to write this book to address the most common concerns, as well as to spread the skills of facial massage.

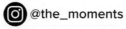 @the_moments

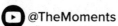 @TheMoments

We hope you enjoyed this Hay House book. If you'd like to receive our online catalog featuring additional information on Hay House books and products, or if you'd like to find out more about the Hay Foundation, please contact:

Hay House LLC, P.O. Box 5100, Carlsbad, CA 92018-5100
(760) 431-7695 or (800) 654-5126
www.hayhouse.com® • www.hayfoundation.org

———

Published in Australia by:
Hay House Australia Publishing Pty Ltd
18/36 Ralph St., Alexandria NSW 2015
Phone: +61 (02) 9669 4299
www.hayhouse.com.au

Published in the United Kingdom by:
Hay House UK Ltd
1st Floor, Crawford Corner,
91–93 Baker Street, London W1U 6QQ
Phone: +44 (0)20 3927 7290
www.hayhouse.co.uk

Published in India by:
Hay House Publishers (India) Pvt Ltd
Muskaan Complex, Plot No. 3,
B-2, Vasant Kunj, New Delhi 110 070
Phone: +91 11 41761620
www.hayhouse.co.in

———

Let Your Soul Grow

Experience life-changing transformation—one video
at a time—with guidance from the world's leading experts.

www.healyourlifeplus.com

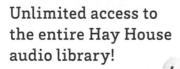

CONNECT WITH

HAY HOUSE

ONLINE

🌐 hayhouse.co.uk   **f** @hayhouse

📷 @hayhouseuk   𝕏 @hayhouseuk

▶ @hayhouseuk   ♪ @hayhouseuk

Find out all about our latest books & card decks • Be the first to know about exclusive discounts • Interact with our authors in live broadcasts • Celebrate the cycle of the seasons with us • Watch free videos from your favourite authors • Connect with like-minded souls

'*The gateways to wisdom and knowledge are always open.*'

Louise Hay